Complimentary and Alternative Medicine in Rheumatology

Guest Editor

SHARON L. KOLASINSKI, MD

RHEUMATIC DISEASE CLINICS OF NORTH AMERICA

www.rheumatic.theclinics.com

February 2011 • Volume 37 • Number 1

SAUNDERS an imprint of ELSEVIER, Inc.

W.B. SAUNDERS COMPANY

A Division of Elsevier Inc.

1600 John F. Kennedy Blvd., Suite 1800 ● Philadelphia, PA 19103-2899

http://www.theclinics.com

RHEUMATIC DISEASE CLINICS OF NORTH AMERICA Volume 37, Number 1

February 2011 ISSN 0889-857X, ISBN 13: 978-1-4557-0502-3

Editor: Rachel Glover

Developmental Editor: Donald Mumford

Rheumatic Disease Clinics of North America (ISSN 0889-857X) is published quarterly by Elsevier Inc., 360 Park Avenue South, New York, NY 10010-1710. Months of issue are February, May, August, and November. Business and editorial offices: 1600 John F. Kennedy Boulevard, Suite 1800, Philadelphia, PA 19103-2899. Periodicals postage paid at New York, NY and additional mailing offices. Subscription prices are USD 282.00 per year for US individuals, USD 501.00 per year for US institutions, USD 139.00 per year for US students and residents, USD 333.00 per year for Canadian individuals, USD 619.00 per year for Canadian institutions, USD 395.00 per year for international individuals, USD 619.00 per year for international institutions, and USD 194.00 per year for Canadian and foreign students/residents. To receive student/resident rate, orders must be accompanied by name of affiliated institution, date of term, and the *signature* of program/residency coordinator on institution letterhead. Orders will be billed at individual rate until proof of status received. Foreign air speed delivery is included in all *Clinics* subscription prices. All prices are subject to change without notice. **POSTMASTER:** Send address changes to *Rheumatic Disease Clinics of North America,* Elsevier Health Sciences Division, Subscription Customer Service, 3251 Riverport Lane, Maryland Heights, MO 63043. **Customer Service: 1-800-654-2452 (US and Canada). From outside of the US and Canada: 314-447-8871. Fax: 314-447-8029. For print support, e-mail: JournalsCustomerService-usa@elsevier.com. For online support, e-mail: JournalsOnline Support-usa@elsevier.com.**

Reprints. For copies of 100 or more of articles in this publication, please contact the Commercial Reprints Department, Elsevier Inc., 360 Park Avenue South, New York, New York, 10010-1710; Tel.: (+1) 212-633-3813, Fax: (+1) 212-462-1935, and E-mail: reprints@elsevier.com.

Rheumatic Disease Clinics of North America is covered in *MEDLINE/PubMed (Index Medicus), Current Contents/Clinical Medicine, Science Citation Index, ISI/BIOMED,* and *EMBASE/Excerpta Medica.*

Printed and bound in the United Kingdom

Transferred to Digital Print 2011

Contributors

GUEST EDITOR

SHARON L. KOLASINSKI, MD, FACP, FACR
Professor of Clinical Medicine, Interim Division Director of Rheumatology, Program
Director, Fellowship in Rheumatology, Division of Rheumatology, University
of Pennsylvania School of Medicine, Philadelphia, Pennsylvania

AUTHORS

SUSAN J. BARTLETT, PhD
Associate Professor of Medicine, Department of Medicine, McGill University, Montreal,
Ontario, Canada; Johns Hopkins Division of Rheumatology, Baltimore, Maryland

SAMIR BHANGLE, MD
Postdoctoral Fellow, Division of Rheumatology, Department of Medicine, University
of Pennsylvania School of Medicine, Philadelphia, Pennsylvania; Department of Medicine,
Saint Barnabas Medical Center, Livingston, New Jersey

DANIEL O. CLEGG, MD
Stevenson Professor of Medicine, Chief, Division of Rheumatology, University of Utah
School of Medicine; George E. Wahlen Department of Veterans Affairs Medical Center,
Salt Lake City, Utah

EDZARD ERNST, MD, PhD, FMedSci, FSB, FRCP, FRCPEd
Professor, Complementary Medicine, Peninsula Medical School, University of Exeter,
Exeter, United Kingdom

STEFFANY HAAZ, PhD
Department of Health, Behavior and Society, Johns Hopkins School of Public Health,
Baltimore, Maryland

ANAN J. HAIJA, MD
Fellow, Division of Rheumatology, Hospital of the University of Pennsylvania, Philadelphia,
Pennsylvania

SHARON L. KOLASINSKI, MD, FACP, FACR
Professor of Clinical Medicine, Interim Division Director of Rheumatology, Program
Director, Fellowship in Rheumatology, Division of Rheumatology, University
of Pennsylvania School of Medicine, Philadelphia, Pennsylvania

SOPHIA LI, MD
Fellow, Division of Rheumatology, Department of Medicine, University of Pennsylvania,
Philadelphia, Pennsylvania

ROBERT MICHELETTI, MD
Resident Physician, Department of Medicine, University of Pennsylvania, Philadelphia,
Pennsylvania

KARLA L. MILLER, MD
Clinical Instructor of Medicine, Division of Rheumatology, University of Utah School of Medicine, Salt Lake City, Utah

RICHARD S. PANUSH, MD, MACP, MACR
Professor of Medicine, Division of Rheumatology, Department of Medicine, Keck School of Medicine, University of Southern California, Los Angeles, California

SHEETAL PATEL, MD
Hospitalist, Hackensack University Medical Center, Hackensack; Department of Medicine, Saint Barnabas Medical Center, Livingston, New Jersey

ADAM PERLMAN, MD, MPH
Chair, Department of Primary Care, Endowed Professor of Complementary and Alternative Medicine, School of Health Related Professions, University of Medicine and Dentistry of New Jersey, Newark; Director, Integrative Medicine, Saint Barnabas Medical Center, Livingston, New Jersey

ROSY RAJBHANDARY, MD
Senior Assistant Resident, Department of Medicine, Saint Barnabas Medical Center, Livingston, New Jersey

STEFFAN W. SCHULZ, MD
Assistant Professor of Clinical Medicine, Division of Rheumatology, Hospital of the University of Pennsylvania, Philadelphia, Pennsylvania

DEEPALI SEN, MD
Senior Assistant Resident, Department of Medicine, Guthrie Clinic, Sayre, Pennsylvania; Department of Medicine, Saint Barnabas Medical Center, Livingston, New Jersey

ROLAND STAUD, MD
Professor of Medicine, Department of Medicine, University of Florida College of Medicine, Gainesville, Florida

KARINE TOUPIN APRIL, OT, PhD
Postdoctoral Fellow, Department of Epidemiology and Community Medicine, Institute of Population Health, University of Ottawa, Ottawa, Ontario, Canada

RISHMA WALJI, ND, PhD
Postdoctoral Fellow, Department of Health, Aging and Society, McMaster University, Hamilton, Ontario, Canada

CHENCHEN WANG, MD, MSc
Associate Professor of Medicine, Division of Rheumatology, Tufts Medical Center, Tufts University School of Medicine, Boston, Massachusetts

LAURA A. YOUNG, MD, PhD
Assistant Professor of Medicine, Division of Endocrinology, Department of Internal Medicine, University of North Carolina School of Medicine, Chapel Hill, North Carolina

Contents

> This article reviews the existing literature on using yoga for arthritis. It includes peer-reviewed research from clinical trials (published from 1980 to 2010) that used yoga as an intervention for arthritis and reported quantitative findings. Eleven studies were identified, including 4 randomized controlled trials (RCTs) and 4 non-RCTs. All trials were small and control groups varied. No adverse events were reported, and attrition was comparable or better than that typical for exercise interventions. Evidence was strongest for reduced disease symptoms (tender/swollen joints, pain) and disability and for improved self-efficacy and mental health. Interventions, research methods, and disease diagnoses were heterogeneous.

> The use of complementary and alternative medicine (CAM) is common among patients with systemic lupus erythematosus (SLE), especially those with active disease who often have poorer quality of life and significant unmet needs. It is important for the rheumatologist to be aware of these therapies and to ask the patient with SLE about their active use or future interest in CAM. Future studies on the effectiveness of the aforementioned therapies will be crucial to find better ways for the rheumatologist to integrate their use into the care of the patient with SLE.

> Over the past decade, there has been an increasing interest in meditation as a mind-body approach, given its potential to alleviate emotional distress and promote improved well being in a variety of populations. The overall purpose of this review is to provide the practicing rheumatologist with an overview of mindfulness and how it can be applied to Western medical treatment plans to enhance both the medical and psychological care of patients.

> In current practice, dietary interventions and over-the-counter dietary supplements, including fish oil, vitamins, and others, comprise a significant proportion of alternate therapy use. The aim of this article is to clarify the appropriate place for the use of fish oil in rheumatologic practice amid the complexities of modern management.

> This article reviews available evidence on complementary and alternative medicine in pediatric rheumatology. Despite its common use in pediatric

rheumatology (34%–92%), there is still uncertainty as to its efficacy and safety. Although results are promising for some treatments such as massage, acupuncture, mind-body interventions (eg, guided imagery and meditative breathing), and some natural health products (eg, calcium supplements and *Tripterygium wilfordii*), there is a need for high-quality trials investigating the long-term effects and underlying mechanisms of these therapies as well as research on their use in this population of patients.

RELATED INTEREST

Primary Care: Clinics in Office Practice, Volume 37, Issue 1 (March 2010)
Integrative Medicine, Part I: Incorporating Complementary/Alternative Modalities
J. Adam Rindfleisch, MD, *Guest Editor*

THE CLINICS ARE NOW AVAILABLE ONLINE!

Access your subscription at:
www.theclinics.com

Preface

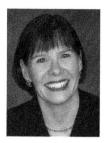

Sharon L. Kolasinski, MD
Guest Editor

It has been almost two decades since the landmark publication of Eisenberg and colleagues[1] brought the magnitude of the use of complementary and alternative medicine (CAM) in the United States to the attention of the traditional medical community. They reported that more than a third of Americans surveyed stated that they had used an "unconventional therapy" to address a health concern in the preceding year. Their groundbreaking epidemiological work was the first of many studies to underscore the widespread and important nature of this phenomenon. In rheumatology and other disciplines, it has subsequently been observed that patients with chronic disease may make use of CAM therapies even more frequently.[2] Initial observations suggested that this might be a phenomenon restricted to those more highly educated, wealthier individuals who could afford such therapies. Subsequent, more broadly based surveys have demonstrated that CAM use is seen across all ages (including children) and all racial and ethnic groups and countries of origin studied.

It has become obvious to many in the traditional medical community that the use of CAM is not diminishing. Patients continue to seek alternatives to what they sometimes perceive as dangerous medications fraught with side effects. However, they also seek practices and treatments that are under their control that might meaningfully affect the way they feel and cope with disease and complement the medical treatments they continue to receive. Both supporters and detractors of CAM recognize that CAM treatments need to be assessed in a scientifically rigorous manner for physicians and their patients to make the most appropriate decisions on their use. Along with this recognition has come a tremendous increase in the number of publications about CAM therapies, including numerous randomized, placebo-controlled trials. It is the purpose of this volume to update the reader on the most recent evidence-based advances in this field. Many had hoped for the emergence of safer, better tolerated pharmaceuticals based on natural products. For the most part, these types of medicines have not emerged. What has evolved over the last several years, however, is a more robust literature on mind-body interventions, particularly in the arena of pain management. Interestingly, this is a group of therapies that rheumatologists are becoming increasingly comfortable recommending.[3] We invite our readers to critically appraise the data presented and

Rheum Dis Clin N Am 37 (2011) ix–x
doi:10.1016/j.rdc.2010.12.001
0889-857X/11/$ – see front matter © 2011 Elsevier Inc. All rights reserved.

rheumatic.theclinics.com

hope that this volume will serve to inform practitioners across many fields about the latest advances and challenges and unanswered questions that remain in complementary and alternative medicine.

Sharon L. Kolasinski, MD
Division of Rheumatology
University of Pennsylvania School of Medicine
8 Penn Tower
34th Street and Civic Center Boulevard
Philadelphia, PA 19104, USA

E-mail address:
Sharon.Kolasinski@uphs.upenn.edu

REFERENCES

1. Eisenberg DM, Kessler RC, Foster C, et al. Unconventional medicine in the United States– Prevalence, costs, and patterns of use. N Engl J Med 1993;328:246–52.
2. Ramos-Remus C, Raut A. Complementary and alternative practices in rheumatology. Best Pract Res Clin Rheumatol 2008;22:741–57.
3. Manek NJ, Crowson CS, Ottenberg AL, et al. What rheumatologists in the United States think of complementary and alternative medicine: results of a national survey. BMC Complement Altern Med 2010;10:5–13.

Perspectives About Complementary and Alternative Medicine in Rheumatology

Rosy Rajbhandary, MD[a], Samir Bhangle, MD[a,b],
Sheetal Patel, MD[a,c], Deepali Sen, MD[a,d],
Adam Perlman, MD, MPH[e,f], Richard S. Panush, MD, MACP, MACR[g,*]

KEYWORDS

- Complementary medicine • Alternative medicine
- Complementary and alternative medicine • Epidemiology
- Demographics • Trends • Appeal • Costs

All who drink of this remedy are cured, except those who die. Thus, it is effective for all but the incurable.

Galen

"I didn't say it was good for you," the king replied. "I said there was nothing like it."

Lewis Carroll. Through The Looking Glass

Perspectives about complementary and alternative medicine (CAM), and CAM therapies, particularly for the rheumatic diseases have changed dramatically over the past several decades.[1–20]

The usage, popularity, and costs of CAM have increased, and the terminology has changed. CAM has become acceptable and perhaps even mainstream. All these

---

[a] Department of Medicine, Saint Barnabas Medical Center, Livingston, NJ, USA
[b] Division of Rheumatology, Department of Medicine, University of Pennsylvania School of Medicine, Philadelphia, PA, USA
[c] Hackensack University Medical Center, 30 Prospect Avenue, Hackensack, NJ 07601, USA
[d] Department of Medicine, Guthrie Clinic, Sayre, PA, USA
[e] Department of Primary Care, School of Health Related Professions, University of Medicine and Dentistry of New Jersey, Newark, NJ 07103, USA
[f] Integrative Medicine, Saint Barnabas Medical Center, Livingston, NJ 07039, USA
[g] Division of Rheumatology, Department of Medicine, Keck School of Medicine, University of Southern California, 2011 Zonal Avenue, HMR 711, Los Angeles, CA 90032, USA
* Corresponding author. Division of Rheumatology, Department of Medicine, Keck School of Medicine, University of Southern California, 2011 Zonal Avenue, HMR 711, Los Angeles, CA 90032.
E-mail address: panush@usc.edu

Rheum Dis Clin N Am 37 (2011) 1–8
doi:10.1016/j.rdc.2010.11.008
0889-857X/11/$ – see front matter © 2011 Elsevier Inc. All rights reserved.
rheumatic.theclinics.com

developments have occurred despite little documentation of efficacy for the treatment of patients with rheumatic diseases. The authors review these aspects of CAM in this article, mindful of the accompanying articles in this issue.

TERMINOLOGY AND DEFINITIONS

It wasn't that long ago that "quackery" denoted what is today termed CAM. Other terms included dubious, unconventional, unproven, questionable, nonstandard, and irregular therapies. Complementary and alternative have been generally used, but not always rigorously or appropriately.[14,16–18] Many today prefer to call this treatment integrative medicine, to reflect the inclusion of evidence-based therapies, regardless of their origin, in conventional practice.[14,16–18] There is even taxonomy for CAM.[21] The authors have favored the terms mainstream and nonmainstream therapies because there have certainly been routine practices that were not supported by evidence or proven safe (ie, tonsillectomy and adenoidectomy, certain arthroscopic and back operations, and even the recent popularity and use of nonsteroidal antiinflammatory drugs [NSAIDs]) and others that are evidence-based but eschewed by given cultures (ie, balneotherapy).[14,16–18,22] However, for purposes of this discussion the authors largely use the term CAM.

WHO USES CAM AND WHY?

Most patients, particularly those with chronic diseases, use CAM. Indeed, the popularity of CAM therapies has led to their incorporation into the medical curriculum at many schools[23,24] and hospitals[25] and to serious efforts to study them scientifically (and the authors have elsewhere praised certain of those individuals[18,19]), to the establishment of a CAM center at the National Institutes of Health (despite opposition from the scientific community), and an increasing aura of legitimacy.[14,16–18]

CAM therapies are widely used throughout the world across geographic, ethnic, social, and economic boundaries. **Table 1** illustrates this generally and for the patients with rheumatic disease specifically.[26–30]

Box 1 summarizes the prevalence of use and the cost of CAM in the United States.[31–33] CAM users tend to be women, well educated, and economically comfortable.[34]

CAM therapies are used for chronic as opposed to life-threatening medical conditions,[35] including cancer, AIDS, gastrointestinal problems, chronic renal failure, depression, and eating disorders. In particular, CAM therapies are frequently used by patients with rheumatologic conditions, such as arthritis, chronic back pain, and other painful musculoskeletal disorders.[36,37] There are now more patient visits to CAM

Table 1 Prevalence of CAM use		
	CAM Use	
Country	**General Population (%)**	**Patients with Rheumatic Diseases (%)**
United States	33–90	28–94
United Kingdom	46	60
Australia	52.2	40–52
Canada	15–32	47–91

Box 1
Contemporary CAM trends in the United States

- About 38% of adults use CAM.
- An expenditure of $34 billion per year is incurred on products and for practitioners.
- There is an annual expenditure of $121.92 per person for CAM.
- CAM constitutes 1.5% of the total health care expenditure and 11.2% of the total out-of-pocket expenditure on health care.

---

practitioners than to primary care physicians in the United States.[38] As has long been documented to be the case, most CAM users do not inform their medical doctors of their use of alternative therapies. Almost 50% of users do so without any professional supervision.[27,39] Patients are likely to choose nonpractitioner-based CAM therapy over practitioner-based CAM therapy.[40]

The use of CAM increases with the number of patients' medical conditions and the number of physician visits. Patients who reported poor health had substantially higher rates of use of CAM therapies than those who perceived themselves to be in better health (52% vs 33%).[38] Studies of patients with specific rheumatologic conditions, such as fibromyalgia, osteoarthritis, and systemic lupus erythematosus, demonstrated that most CAM users were generally people with chronic disease, poorer functional status, and higher levels of pain.[40]

Patients use CAM therapies because these therapies (1) are consonant with their lifestyle and/or belief system, (2) produce a sense of a holistic approach to medical care, (3) are perceived to be safer and more natural than prescription drugs, (4) help them to achieve greater control over their illness and its management and reflecttheir rejection of or dissatisfaction with conventional medical care (for many reasons including perceived impersonal skills of practitioners, cost and toxicities of mainstream therapies, and uncertainties about outcomes).[14,16–18,41] Practitioners of CAM are often considered more available, more empathetic, more caring, as investing more time with patients, and as conveying more confidence and optimism about outcomes than regular physicians. Studies have shown that patients preferring CAM tended to be more psychologically distressed and considered their health poorer than that of others. Most patients use CAM to complement conventional care rather than to substitute for it.[14,16–18,42]

TRENDS

The frequency of use of the different CAM modalities has changed over the past several decades. The 1960s saw a growth in the use of diets, megavitamins and self-help groups. The 1970s featured an increase in the use of biofeedback, energy healing, folk remedies, herbal medicine, homeopathy, hypnosis, and spiritual healing and imagery. In the 1980s, massage and naturopathy became popular and interest in yoga decreased. Aromatherapy, energy healing, herbal medicine, massage, and yoga became more prevalent in the 1990s.[43] The usage of CAM has remained stable since.[37,44–46]

Although it is beyond the scope of this article to review all CAM therapies used by patients with rheumatic diseases, some of the major modalities and the authors' assessments of their efficacy have been summarized in **Box 2**. (The authors appreciate that others may interpret the available evidence differently.)

Box 2
Efficacy of various CAM modalities for patients with rheumatic diseases

Therapies known not to be a clinical benefit

  Apheresis

  Antibiotics (except minocycline for rheumatoid arthritis)

  Copper bracelets

  Glucosamine+

Therapies not studied

  Shark cartilage

  Cetyl myristeolate

  Methylsulfonylmethane

Therapies with preliminary, incomplete, or inconsistent evidence of benefit but not (yet) adequately studied

  Ginger

  Ayurveda

  Yoga

  Homeopathy

  Photopheresis

  Magnets

  Pulsed electromagnetic fields

  Oral collagen

  S-adenosylmethionine

  Venoms

  Diet and nutritional regimens

  Herbal therapies

  Prayer/distant healing

  Zinc

  Manipulation

  Diacerhein

  Massage therapy

Therapies generally accepted of proven value

  Spa/balneotherapy

  Exercise

  Mind-body therapies

  Fish/botanic oils

  Acupuncture

Data from Panush RS. Questionable remedies. Up-To-Date In Medicine. Schur PH, Section editor for rheumatology, Rose B, Editor-in-Chief. Wellesley (MA); 1997 (updated quarterly, revised annually).

Box 3
Principles of complementary and alternative therapies for rheumatic diseases

- If it sounds too good to be true, it is.
- If you have not read about it in the scientific literature, it is not validated.
- There are no secrets in good science or good medicine.
- There have been no "breakthrough," important advances in rheumatology from complementary and alternative medicine.
- The question regarding trying complementary and alternative therapies should not be why not but why?
- Discuss complementary and alternative therapies with patients.[58]
- We believe in science, scientific methods, and a single high standard of good evidence-based medicine for all patients.

Data from Panush RS. Questionable remedies. Up-To-Date In Medicine. Schur PH, Section editor for rheumatology, Rose B, Editor-in-Chief. Wellesley (MA); 1997 (updated quarterly, revised annually); and Panush RS. Shift happens. Complementary and alternative medicine for rheumatologists. J Rheumatol 2002;29:656–8.

SAFETY OF COMPLEMENTARY AND ALTERNATIVE THERAPIES

The misconception that CAM therapies are natural and harmless is prevalent in patients using them. However, CAM may or may not be so.[38,47] CAM products can be harmful. Patients have suffered, and a few, fortunately rarely, have died, of infections, injections, and contaminants of CAM modalities, such as arsenic, lead, mercury, caffeine, analgesics, phenylbutazone, steroids, NSAIDs, and ephedrine.[14,16–18,48–52] There are potential interactions between many herbal therapies and conventional medications, some clinically important, which are not always recognized. There are also direct adverse effects of certain CAM therapies, such as bleeding, pain, hematoma, rarely pneumothorax from acupuncture[53] and headache, local discomfort, dizziness, and a rare cerebrovascular accident from manipulation.[54] Some patients received up to 19 remedies, discontinued their formal treatment 11 times, visited CAM providers up to 180 times, and spent the equivalent of 1.3 days' wages on CAM, all of these in one year.[55] Also, there are the obvious consequences of patients not communicating with their rheumatologist (or other physicians) about CAM use.[14,16–18,56,57] The authors do not recommend the use of CAM therapies except for evidence-based indications of anticipated clinical benefit.

SUMMARY

CAM treatments are considered nonmainstream therapies. Their popularity and widespread usage reflects the inadequacies of the current understanding and management of rheumatic and musculoskeletal (and other) diseases, despite significant progress. The authors believe, like Bertram Russell, that "what science cannot tell us, mankind cannot know"; better science in the future will relegate certain CAM therapies to the margins of medicine or to history and perhaps see the adoption of others into mainstream medicine. Despite the recent increased interest in CAM, particularly for rheumatic diseases, perhaps derived in part from the hope of identifying new and useful approaches, few clinically important contributions have emerged thus far. The authors therefore developed recommendations regarding CAM treatments for their patients, which are reflected in **Box 3**.

REFERENCES

1. Panush RS. Controversial arthritis remedies. Bull Rheum Dis 1985;34:1–10.
2. Panush RS, Endo LP. Diet and unproven remedies. In: Katz W, editor. Diagnosis and management of rheumatic disease. Philadelphia: Lippincott; 1988. p. 964–70. Chapter 96.
3. Panush RS. Non-traditional remedies. In: Schumacher HR, editor. Primer on the rheumatic diseases. 9th edition. Atlanta (GA): Arthritis Foundation; 1988. p. 311–5. Chapter 81.
4. Panush RS. Nutritional therapy for rheumatic disease [editorial]. Ann Intern Med 1987;106:619–21.
5. Panush RS. Arthritis, food allergy, diets, and nutrition. In: McCarty DJ, editor. Arthritis and allied conditions-a textbook of rheumatology. Philadelphia: Lea and Febiger; 1988. p. 1010–4. Chapter 65.
6. Panush RS. Nutrition and rheumatic diseases. Rheum Dis Clin 1991;17:197–456, VII–XIV.
7. Panush RS. Diet and arthritis. Position paper for American College of Rheumatology, 1990.
8. Panush RS. Reflections on unproven remedies. Rheum Dis Clin 1993;19:201–6.
9. Panush RS. Is there a role for diet or other questionable therapies in managing rheumatic diseases? Bull Rheum Dis 1993;42:1–4.
10. Panush RS. Alternative medicine: science or superstition? [editorial]. J Rheumatol 1994;21:8–9.
11. Panush RS. Diet and rheumatic disease. Update. In: Kelley WN, Harris ED, Sledge CB, et al, editors. Textbook of rheumatology. Orlando (FL): WB Saunders Co; 1994. p. 1–10.
12. Panush RS. Questionable remedies. In: Klippel JH, Weyand C, Wortman B, editors. Primer on the rheumatic diseases. 11th edition. Atlanta (GA): Arthritis Foundation; 1997. p. 450–2. Chapter 57.
13. Panush RS. Questionable interventions for rheumatic diseases. In: Wegener S, Belza B, Gall E, editors. Primer on clinical care in rheumatic disease. American College of Rheumatology; 1996. p. 107–9.
14. Panush RS. Questionable remedies. Up-To-Date In Medicine: Schur PH, Section editor for rheumatology, Rose B, Editor-in-Chief. Wellesley (MA); 1997 (updated quarterly, revised annually).
15. Panush RS. American College of Rheumatology Position statement: "complementary" and "alternative" therapies for rheumatic diseases. 1998.
16. Panush RS. Complementary and alternative therapies for rheumatic disease. Rheum Dis Clin 1999.
17. Panush RS, Perlman A. Complementary and alternative medicine. Physician Information and Education Resource (PIER) project. Section editors. Philadelphia: American College of Physicians; 2000.
18. Panush RS. Shift happens. Complementary and alternative medicine for rheumatologists. J Rheumatol 2002;29:656–8.
19. Perlman A. Complementary and alternative medicine. Med Clin North Am 2002;86:xi–202.
20. Perlman AI, Sabina A, Williams AL, et al. Massage therapy for osteoarthritis of the knee: a randomized controlled trial. Arch Intern Med 2006;166:2533–8.
21. Kaptchuk TJ, Eisenberg DM. Varieties of healing. 2: a taxonomy of unconventional healing practices. Ann Intern Med 2001;135:196–204.

22. Astin JA, Marie A, Pelletier KR, et al. A review of the incorporation of complementary and alternative medicine by mainstream physicians. Arch Intern Med 1998; 158:2303–10.
23. Perlman A, Stagnarro-Green A. Developing a complementary, alternative, and integrative medicine course: one medical school's experience. J Altern Complement Med 2010;16:601–5.
24. Wetzel MS, Eisenberg DM, Kaptchuk TJ. Courses involving complementary and alternative medicine at US medical schools. JAMA 1998;280:784–7.
25. Press release and statements. Latest survey shows more hospitals offering complementary and alternative medicine services. Washington, DC: American Hospital Association; 2008.
26. Ramos-Remus C, Raut A. Complementary and alternative practices in rheumatology. Best Pract Res Clin Rheumatol 2008;22:741–57.
27. Rao JK. Complementary and alternative medicine for arthritis. N C Med J 2007; 68:453–5.
28. Xue CC, Zhang AL, Lin V, et al. Complementary and alternative medicine use in Australia: a national population-based survey. J Altern Complement Med 2007; 13:643–50.
29. MacLennan AH, Myers SP, Taylor AW. The continuing use of complementary and alternative medicine in South Australia: costs and beliefs in 2004. Med J Aust 2006;184:27–31.
30. Esmail N. Complementary and alternative medicine in Canada: trends in use and public attitudes, 1997–2006. Public policy sources, number 87. Vancouver (British Columbia), Canada: Fraser Institute; 2007.
31. Barnes PM, Bloom B, Nahin RL. Complementary and alternative medicine use among adults and children: United States, 2007. Natl Health Stat Report 2008; 12:1–23.
32. Nahin RL, Barnes PM, Stussman BJ, et al. Costs of Complementary and Alternative Medicine (CAM) and Frequency of Visits to CAM Practitioners: United States, 2007. National health statistics reports; no 18. Hyattsville (MD): National Center for Health Statistics; 2009. Available at: http://www.nccam.nih.gov/news/camstats.htm. Accessed November 8, 2010.
33. Fisher P, Ward A. Complementary medicine in Europe. BMJ 1994;309:107–10.
34. Nahin RL, Dahlhamer JM, Taylor BL, et al. Health behaviors and risk factors in those who use complementary and alternative medicine. BMC Public Health 2007;7(147):217.
35. Quandt SA, Chen H, Grzywacz JG, et al. Use of complementary and alternative medicine by persons with arthritis: result of the national health interview survey. Arthritis Rheum 2005;53:748–55.
36. Coopes MJ, Anderson RA, Egeler RM, et al. Alternative therapies for the treatment of childhood cancer. N Engl J Med 1998;339:846.
37. Saydah S, Eberhardt M. Use of complementary and alternative medicine among adults with chronic diseases: United States 2002. J Altern Complement Med 2006;12:805–12.
38. Eisenberg DM, Kessler RC, Foster C, et al. Unconventional medicine in the United States– prevalance, costs and patterns of use. N Engl J Med 1993;328: 246–52.
39. Rao JK, Kroenke K, Mihaliak KA, et al. Rheumatolgy patients' use of complementary therapies: results from a one-year longitudinal study. Arthritis Rheum 2003; 49:619–25.

40. Rao JK, Kroenke K, Mihaliak KA, et al. Use of complementary therapies for arthritis among patients of rheumatologists. Ann Intern Med 1999;131:409–16.
41. Astin JA. Why patients use alternative medicine: results of a national study. JAMA 1998;279:1548.
42. Chandola A, Young Y, McAlister J, et al. Use of complementary therapies by patients attending musculoskeletal clinics. J Rheumatol 1999;26:2468–74.
43. Kessler RC, Davis RB, Foster DF, et al. Long term trends in the use of complementary and alternative medical therapies in the United States. Ann Intern Med 2001;35:262–8.
44. Eisenberg D, Davis R, Ettner S, et al. Trends in alternative medicine use in the United States, 1990–1997. JAMA 1998;280:1569–75.
45. Barnes P, Powell-Griner E, McFann K, et al. Complementary and alternative medicine use among adults: United States, 2002. from Vital and Health Statistics. Adv Data 2004;343:1–19.
46. Tindle H, Davis R, Phillips R, et al. Trends in use of complementary and alternative medicine by US adults 1997–2002. Altern Ther Health Med 2005;11:42–9.
47. Boisset M, Fittzcharles MA. Alternative medicine use by rheumatic patients in a universal health care setting. J Rheum 1994;21:148–52.
48. Huang WF, Wen KC, Hsiao ML. Adulteration by synthetic therapeutic substances of traditional Chinese medicines in Taiwan. J Clin Pharmacol 1997;37:344–50.
49. Gertner E, Marshall PS, Filandrinos D, et al. Complications resulting from the use of Chinese herbal medications containing undeclared prescription drugs. Arthritis Rheum 1995;38:614–7.
50. Goldman JA. Chinese herbal medicine: camouflaged prescription anti-inflammatory drugs, corticosteroids, and lead. Arthritis Rheum 1991;34:1207.
51. Ries CA, Sahud MA. Agranulocytosis caused by Chinese herbal medicines: dangers of medications containing aminopyrine and phenylbutazone. JAMA 1975;231:352–5.
52. Ko RJ. Adulterants in Asian patent medicines. N Engl J Med 1998;339:847.
53. Melchart D, Weidenhammer W, Streng A, et al. Prospective investigation of adverse effects of acupuncture in 97,733 patients. Arch Intern Med 2004;164:104–5.
54. Stevinson C, Ernst E. Risks associated with spinal manipulation. Am J Med 2002;112:566–71.
55. Ramos-Remus C, Gamez-Nava JI, Gonzalez-Lopez L, et al. Use of non-conventional therapies by patients with rheumatic diseases in Guadalajara, Mexico: prevalence, beliefs and expectations. Arthritis Care Res 1998;11:411–8.
56. Barnes J, Mills SY, Abott NC, et al. Different standards for reporting ADRs to herbal remedies and conventional OTC medicines: face-to-face interviews with 515 users of herbal remedies. Br J Clin Pharmacol 1998;45:496–500.
57. Barnes J. Pharmacovigilance of herbal medicines: a UK perspective. Drug Saf 2003;26:829–51.
58. Perlman A, Eisenberg D, Panush RS. Talking with patients about complementary and alternative therapies. Rheum Dis Clin 1999;25:815–22.

Effectiveness of CAM Therapy: Understanding the Evidence

Roland Staud, MD

KEYWORDS

• Efficacy • Treatment • Complementary Medicine

Complementary and alternative medicine (CAM) was defined by the National Center for Complementary and Alternative Medicine as a group of diverse medical and health care systems, practices, and products that are currently not integrated into conventional medicine.[1] Patients with chronic conditions, including pain, who often experience only limited symptom relief with traditional medical therapies, show high rates of CAM use.[2,3] Several literature reviews of nonpharmacologic interventions for chronic pain syndromes have examined the use of such therapies, including cognitive-behavioral therapy (CBT), exercise, acupuncture, spinal manipulation, diet, herbal supplements, massage, and other CAM therapies.[4–11] Using widely accepted criteria for such types of reviews,[12] evidence of clinical effectiveness was shown only for exercise and CBT. The results for acupuncture interventions for chronic pain syndromes were inconclusive.

Historically, CAM is not routinely prescribed by practitioners of conventional Western medicine, taught in medical schools, or reimbursed by third-party payers. Much of this situation is because research on the therapeutic effects of CAM is still in its infancy. The National Institutes of Health has classified CAM in 5 ways: (1) alternative medical systems, such as traditional Chinese medicine (including acupuncture), naturopathic medicine, Ayurvedic medicine, and homeopathy; (2) biologic-based therapies, including herbal, special dietary, and individual biologic treatments not accepted by the US Food and Drug Administration (FDA); (3) energy therapies, such as Reiki, therapeutic touch, magnet therapy, Qi Gong, and intercessory prayer; (4) manipulative and body-based systems, for example, chiropractic, osteopathy, and massage; and (5) mind-body interventions, such as meditation, biofeedback, hypnotherapy, and the relaxation response.[13] This review focuses on the effectiveness of CAM therapies for chronic musculoskeletal pains, with emphasis on the role of specific and nonspecific analgesic mechanisms, including placebo.

Department of Medicine, University of Florida College of Medicine, Gainesville, FL 32610-0221, USA
E-mail address: staudr@ufl.edu

Rheum Dis Clin N Am 37 (2011) 9–17
doi:10.1016/j.rdc.2010.11.009
0889-857X/11/$ – see front matter © 2011 Elsevier Inc. All rights reserved.

WHAT IS THE EVIDENCE FOR EFFECTIVENESS OF CAM THERAPY?

Much of the criticism of CAM therapies is based on the claim that, in contrast to conventional medicine, CAM is not evidence based. However, most of this criticism depends on what experts consider acceptable evidence.[14] Treatment recommendations are often considered evidence-based after trials have found specific interventions to be superior to placebo controls or at least as equally effective as established therapies. Most of the time randomized, double-blind, placebo-controlled studies are accepted as best evidence.[15] However, evidence is a complex construct, with different meanings depending on the topic of study. Because circumstances differ considerably, not only randomized and nonrandomized trials but also qualitative studies may be necessary to detect the effects of a specific treatment. In every trial multiple different factors may affect the study outcomes, including measurement errors, regression to the mean, and the natural course of the disease studied. In addition, nonspecific treatment effects need to be considered, including placebo effects (often related to expectations and desires), attention of health care providers, as well as unspecific effects such as healing. There are also specific factors of treatment that affect biologic mechanisms. High-level evidence can be obtained only if the final analysis combines all of these factors.[16–18] Furthermore, the notion to compare only active intervention with placebo may result in wrong conclusions[19]: just because the effects of a specific treatment might be indistinguishable from a placebo and therefore could be considered ineffective, may not preclude this therapy from being more efficacious than another treatment used for the same purpose. The latter treatment might even have shown greater effectiveness than placebo in a controlled trial. One explanation for this paradox is that not all placebo effects are of similar magnitude. Therefore judging treatment efficacy based only on calculations of difference scores between active and placebo treatment may be too restrictive. Placebo effects can vary considerably between studies and thus some placebo interventions might be more therapeutic than well-established specific treatments.

MAGNITUDE OF PLACEBO EFFECTS

Although placebos have been used for many different types of interventions, this discussion focuses on the placebo effect on pain. Placebo effects are not measured in randomized controlled trials (RCTs) but are only controlled for. To measure placebo effects a natural history condition is needed, because the differential between the efficacy of a natural history condition and placebo condition represents the placebo effect. The magnitude of placebo analgesia may range from none to large responses. Furthermore, it is well known that there are placebo responders and nonresponders. In 1955, Beecher[20] estimated that approximately 30% of patients responded to placebo treatments for pain. However, this study was flawed because it lacked a no-treatment group. Subsequently, several well-executed studies of placebo analgesia that used no-treatment groups[21–23] identified between 27% and 56% of participants as responders to placebo treatment. It is well known that placebo effects can differ across studies, and this difference is mostly because of changes of experimental conditions. Using standard placebo instructions, several studies have reported small placebo analgesic effects.[24–28] However, when only placebo responders were analyzed the average magnitude of analgesia more than doubled.[22] In addition, experimental manipulations used to induce placebo analgesia seem to strongly influence the magnitude of the patients' responses, specifically after strong verbal suggestions.[29,30] Verbal suggestions that trigger expectations of analgesia induce larger placebo responses than those inducing ambiguous expectations. This point was best illustrated by studies using standard verbal instructions ("You will receive either placebo or a painkiller") or strong placebo suggestions ("The treatment you are going to receive has been found to powerfully reduce pain in some patients").[31] Greater analgesic effects were obtained with enhanced placebo instructions compared with regular instructions. These placebo studies show that subtle differences in instruction sets may have a substantial effect on the magnitude of the response. Furthermore, previous pain experiences can either increase or decrease the magnitude of placebo analgesia, specifically when pain reductions or pain increases are expected by the participants.[32] These results indicate that placebo effects may depend on cognitive factors, thus explaining at least some of the variability of placebo responses observed among studies.

OTHER FACTORS THAT CONTRIBUTE TO UNSPECIFIC TREATMENT EFFECTS

Therapeutic regimens often provide not only specific but also nonspecific benefits, which may include more than only placebo effects. Such nonspecific effects can be separated into the patient's response to observation and assessment (also called the Hawthorne effect), the patient's response to the administration of a dummy treatment (placebo effect), and the patient's response to the patient-physician interaction (healing effect).[33–36] When these distinct factors were manipulated in a placebo trial of patients with irritable bowel syndrome (IBS), they were found to produce progressive improvements resembling a graded dose escalation.[37] Specifically, an enhanced relationship with a practitioner, together with a placebo treatment, was identified as the most robust effect, followed by placebo treatment with only limited interaction with physicians, which nevertheless was superior to being on a waiting list. The magnitude of nonspecific effects for some patients was large and clinically significant, resulting in a substantial decrease of symptom severity. Moreover, this effect could be maintained for up to 6 weeks. More than 60% of patients reported adequate relief, which is comparable with the responder rate of currently used drug treatments of IBS.[38,39] These results indicate that factors such as warmth, empathy, duration of interaction, and the communication of positive expectation might significantly affect clinical outcome. Future investigations will have to determine the relative importance of each of these elements of the patient-practitioner relationship.

MAGNITUDE OF SPECIFIC AND UNSPECIFIC TREATMENT FACTORS

Current medical concepts are dominated by biomedical models, which have helped in explaining the pathogenesis of acute diseases and have provided the rationale for evidence-based interventions. However, these medical models have failed many patients with chronic illnesses, most of which involve multiple interconnected systems. To better characterize their pathologic conditions biopsychosocial models have increasingly been used. The relevant illnesses include, but are not limited to, systemic lupus erythematosus, rheumatoid arthritis, fibromyalgia, chronic fatigue syndrome, IBS, and headaches. Although some models seem to perform well to characterize these illnesses their treatments often have been unsatisfactory. RCTs have been conducted for the treatment of most of these illnesses on the premise that effectiveness can be assumed only if there is efficacy, and that efficacy is dependent on superiority of the active treatment to placebo. Thus RCTs usually use placebo interventions to control for nonspecific effects of therapy,[40] which include but are not limited to regression to the mean and the natural course of the disease under study. Although the final analysis of RCTs almost always uses statistical comparisons of specific effects with placebo controls, the effect size of nonspecific treatment effects is generally not reported despite often being larger than specific effects.[41]

The important role of unspecific effects embedded in many therapies is emphasized by the high correlation observed between specific and unspecific treatment effects. Several studies reported strong correlations between therapeutic effects of placebo and active treatment, which accounted for most of the variance (60%–90%).[41–43] These high correlations are not surprising, because unspecific effects are operative in all treatment conditions. On the other hand, some specific study treatments may surreptitiously become more efficacious than placebo because treatment side effects may attenuate the study blind and interfere with allocation concealment.[44,45] Such unblinding may raise expectations related to treatment outcomes and simultaneously increase the magnitude of effects of active interventions. To avoid such nonspecific effects, all clinical trials need to query participants at the final visit about their beliefs on trial assignments. The fact that unspecific effects seem to explain more than 50% of the variance in many RCTs is a clue that the commonality of factors within trials may be greater than their difference (ie, nonspecific treatment effects can contribute more to final outcomes than specific ones). A detailed analysis of multiple treatment studies identified several factors as responsible for the variability of therapeutic responses in placebo groups.[43] It suggested that unspecific treatment effects are especially high in treatment studies of long duration and in prevention trials. Of all factors examined prevention trials seemed to elicit the strongest placebo effects.[43] Furthermore, the same analysis showed that placebo variability differed for different illnesses. In general, improvement rates in placebo groups were greater in studies of antidepressants and antianxiety medications for affective disorders, but lower for substance-withdrawal studies and trials of antiepileptics. This variance in placebo efficacy across different studies raises suspicions that publication bias may have been involved.[46] Because publication of clinical trials is strongly biased in favor of interventions that outperform unspecific treatment effects,[47] the results of unpublished studies with negative outcomes were considered to be necessary for calculations of placebo variances. However, statistical simulations showed that publication bias alone was unlikely to account for the variability of observed placebo effects.[43] Thus placebo variability in clinical trials is affected not only by methodological factors,[48] but also by unspecific effects like Hawthorne effects, conditioning, and healing response.

OBTAINING THE EVIDENCE

The double-blind RCT, in which neither the trial investigators nor trial participants know who is receiving the active treatment, has long been accepted as the gold standard for determining statistical and clinical efficacy. The use of blinding, random allocation, and control groups is believed to help determine whether the treatment itself or other factors are responsible for the observed effects. RCTs are used by regulators to evaluate the effectiveness and safety of treatments, as well as a way to ensure human experimentation takes place in controlled environments that are also subject to regulatory oversight. Drug manufacturers are required by the FDA to show evidence of the safety and efficacy of new drugs through adequate and well-controlled trials. The value of RCTs has become accepted by clinicians and regulators as a way to avoid anecdotal claims of therapeutic efficacy. Although most RCTs are either conducted or funded by the pharmaceutical industry, the core methodology of RCTs is considered safe against bias. Despite methodological deficits of some RCTs to assess the efficacy of complex treatment strategies these failures are often used as evidence for the need to improve but not radically change trial designs and analysis. CAM therapies specifically are frequently criticized for their inadequate trial designs and analytical techniques. Often, when treatment effects are difficult to measure quantitatively, as with many CAM therapies, new or additional methods of evaluation are necessary to better gauge treatment responses. Another problem with RCTs is that their results are often accepted by health care providers because of statistical significance despite lack of clinical usefulness. Such limitations of RCTs are especially apparent with CAM therapies and psychiatric treatments, the effects of which are often difficult to measure.

The difficulty in measuring the effects of CAM treatments can be seen at every stage of trial design. To determine whether a participant is eligible for enrolment in a CAM trial, one first has to ascertain whether the patient has the required disorder, and determine its level of severity. This aim is a challenge for CAM practitioners, whose methods of diagnosing patients can vary widely. To address this problem, rating scales have been developed to code and categorize behaviors and other relevant factors. Often composite scores are used for capturing mood, sleep, physical and sexual function, and so on. Subsequently, such scores are used to quantify a patient's illness. The challenge for CAM research is proving that the benefits of a treatment are significantly different compared with placebo. To address the problem of placebo responders, researchers have used practices aimed at eliminating such subjects from research trials. One frequently used strategy involves the use of single-blind placebo run-in periods in which all participants unknowingly receive placebo. Subsequently, placebo responders are removed from the trial. However, use of such screening methods raises concerns about the applicability of the study results to the general population. Overall, run-in periods and other tactics adopted by researchers to meet regulatory requirements for statistical evidence of efficacy do not seem to live up to initial hopes and expectations.

FUTURE PERSPECTIVES

Because most research to date has focused on the efficacy of individual treatment modalities, new approaches for the evaluation of CAM therapies are needed. One promising approach is focused on whole-system research (WSR).[49] Whole systems have been defined as "approaches to health care in which practitioners apply bodies of knowledge and associated practices to maximize the patients' capacity to achieve mental and physical balance and restore their own health, using individualized, nonreductionist approaches to diagnosis and treatment."[50] Instead of specific treatments the practitioner-patient relationship and therapeutic environment play a central role.

Assessing the efficacy of whole-system treatments is complex because all key components of well-being need to be included.[33–36] As mentioned earlier, RCTs are widely accepted as the gold standard for assessing clinical efficacy, but have significant limitations, especially when applied to CAM therapies. Despite good internal validity, RCTs often have poor external validity (generalizability). CAM therapies frequently rely on individualized diagnostic and therapeutic methods unique to different healing techniques, thus making standardized diagnostic approaches difficult or inappropriate. Furthermore, randomization may also become difficult or even impossible, because many whole-system treatments depend on the willingness of the patients to participate in the healing process. The important contributions of patient perceptions and expectations about therapeutic interventions require careful assessments. Thus the specific requirements of RCTs may be inappropriate for this therapeutic process and its outcome.[51] Therefore the Institute of Medicine suggested adaptations of RCTs and other study designs, such as observational studies, to better assess the effectiveness of CAM.[52] Some variations of the classic RCT design that may be appropriate for the evaluation of CAM therapies include:

1. Pragmatic trials for assessments of individualized treatments. Although all participants are randomized to different treatments, the interventions are based on usual medical care. Using such a pragmatic approach in a large RCT the investigators compared individualized usage of acupuncture for chronic headache in general practice.[53] Experimental control was maintained by randomizing participants to treatment groups, but the intervention was intended to represent real-world care.
2. Factorial designs that can compare single treatments with treatment combinations. This approach controls for multiple interaction effects between treatments. For example, the UK back pain exercise and manipulation (BEAM) trial evaluated the effectiveness of several manipulations to best care in the treatment of back pain in general practice.[54]
3. Preference trials may represent a useful approach for CAM trials if patient randomization is difficult or inappropriate. This design may be especially relevant for CAM trials if a patient's preferences are strongly influenced by perceived treatment effectiveness.[55,56] In such trials, participants with no treatment preferences are randomized to the available treatment options but those with preferences receive their preferred treatment, allowing for the assessment of the interaction between treatment preference and treatment outcome.[56]
4. n-of-1 trials can be ideal for the assessment of individual treatment responses. In n-of-1 trials participants are crossed over between experimental and control conditions (ie, placebo or standard therapy).[57] However, information from n-of-1 trials is limited, because such trials can provide only individual level data and thus lack generalizability.[58]

SUMMARY

The challenge of assessing often small effects of complex therapies in diverse populations is not unique to CAM. It also applies to conventional medicine, specifically to symptom-based treatments such as mental health and pain therapy. WSR may provide information about unspecific treatment effects inherent to almost all medical care. Some of these unspecific effects include placebo effects, which are relevant to both CAM and conventional medicine. RCTs are widely accepted as the gold standard for testing specific treatment effects in allopathic medicine, but no similar trial standard exists for symptom-based therapies, including CAM. Thus more advanced CAM trial designs are needed. However, besides measuring specific as well as unspecific treatment effects, new trial designs also need to take into account the influence of ethnic, social, and religious backgrounds of study participants on trial outcomes.

REFERENCES

1. [Anon]. CAM definition. National Center for Complementary and Alternative Medicine; 2010. Available at: http://nccam.nih.gov/health/whatiscam/#I. Accessed November 17, 2010.
2. Barnes P, Powell-Griner E, McFann K, et al. Complementary and alternative medicine use among adults: United States, 2002. Advance data from vital and health statistics 343, 1–20. 2004. Hyattsville (MD): National Center for Health Statistics.

3. Pioro-Boisset M, Esdaile JM, Fitzcharles MA. Alternative medicine use in fibromyalgia syndrome. Arthritis Care Res 1996;9(1):13–7.
4. Ernst E. Prevalence of use of complementary/alternative medicine: a systematic review. Bull World Health Organ 2000;78(2):252–7.
5. Sim J, Adams N. Systematic review of randomized controlled trials of nonpharmacological interventions for fibromyalgia. Clin J Pain 2002;18(5):324–36.
6. Rossy LA, Buckelew SP, Dorr N, et al. A meta-analysis of fibromyalgia treatment interventions. Ann Behav Med 1999;21(2):180–91.
7. Ernst E. Complementary and alternative medicine for fibromyalgia. In: Wallace DJ, Clauw DJ, editors. Fibromyalgia and other central pain syndromes. Philadelphia: Lippincott William & Wilkins; 2005. p. 383–408.
8. Mayhew E, Ernst E. Acupuncture for fibromyalgia - a systemic review of randomized clinical trials. Rheumatology 2007;46:801–4.
9. Ernst E. Complementary treatments in rheumatic diseases. Rheum Dis Clin North Am 2008;34(2):455–67.
10. Perry R, Terry R, Ernst E. A systematic review of homoeopathy for the treatment of fibromyalgia. Clin Rheumatol 2010;29(5):457–64.
11. Crofford LJ, Appleton BE. Complementary and alternative therapies for fibromyalgia. Curr Rheumatol Rep 2001;3(2):147–56.
12. Jadad AR, Cook DJ, Jones A, et al. Methodology and reports of systematic reviews and meta-analyses: a comparison of Cochrane reviews with articles published in paper-based journals. JAMA 1998;280(3):278–80.
13. [Anon]. What is complementary and alternative medicine? NCCAM Publication D156. National Center for Complementary and Alternative Medicine. Available at: http://nccam.nih.gov/health/whatiscam/. Accessed November 17, 2010.
14. Singh S, Ernst E. Trick or treatment? Alternative medicine on trial. New York: Bantam Press; 2008.
15. Guyatt GH, Oxman AD, Kunz R, et al. Going from evidence to recommendations. BMJ 2008;336(7652):1049–51.
16. Walach H, Falkenberg T, Fonnebo V, et al. Circular instead of hierarchical: methodological principles for the evaluation of complex interventions. BMC Med Res Methodol 2006;6:29.
17. Coulter ID. Evidence summaries and synthesis: necessary but insufficient approach for determining clinical practice of integrated medicine? Integr Cancer Ther 2006;5(4):282–6.
18. Jonas WB, Beckner W, Coulter I. Proposal for an integrated evaluation model for the study of whole systems health care in cancer. Integr Cancer Ther 2006; 5(4):315–9.
19. Walach H. The efficacy paradox in randomized controlled trials of CAM and elsewhere: beware of the placebo trap. J Altern Complement Med 2001; 7(3):213–8.
20. Beecher HK. The powerful placebo. JAMA 1955;159:1602–6.
21. Levine JD, Gordon NC, Bornstein JC, et al. Role of pain in placebo analgesia. Proc Natl Acad Sci U S A 1979;76(7):3528–31.
22. Benedetti F. The opposite effects of the opiate antagonist naloxone and the cholecystokinin antagonist proglumide on placebo analgesia. Pain 1996; 64(3):535–43.
23. Petrovic P, Kalso E, Petersson KM, et al. Placebo and opioid analgesia – imaging a shared neuronal network. Science 2002;295(5560):1737–40.
24. Amanzio M, Pollo A, Maggi G, et al. Response variability to analgesics: a role for non-specific activation of endogenous opioids. Pain 2001;90(3):205–15.

25. Benedetti F, Amanzio M, Maggi G. Potentiation of placebo analgesia by proglumide. Lancet 1995;346(8984):1231.
26. Gracely RH, Dubner R, Wolskee PJ, et al. Placebo and naloxone can alter post-surgical pain by separate mechanisms. Nature 1983;306(5940):264–5.
27. Levine JD, Gordon NC. Influence of the method of drug administration on analgesic response. Nature 1984;312(5996):755–6.
28. Price DD, Riley JL, Wade JB. Psychophysical approaches to measurement of the dimensions and stages of pain. In: Turk DC, Melzack R, editors. Handbook of pain assessment. 2nd edition. New York: Guilford Press; 2001. p. 53–75.
29. Vase L, Price DD, Verne GN, et al. The contribution of changes in expected pain levels and desire for relief to placebo analgesia. In: Price DD, Bushnell MC, editors, Psychological methods of pain control: basic science and clinical perspectives, 29. Seattle (WA): IASP Press; 2004. p. 207–32.
30. Vase L, Robinson ME, Verne GN, et al. Increased placebo analgesia over time in irritable bowel syndrome (IBS) patients is associated with desire and expectation but not endogenous opioid mechanisms. Pain 2005;115(3):338–47.
31. Vase L, Robinson ME, Verne GN, et al. The contributions of suggestion, desire, and expectation to placebo effects in irritable bowel syndrome patients–an empirical investigation. Pain 2003;105(1–2):17–25.
32. Colloca L, Benedetti F, Pollo A. Repeatability of autonomic responses to pain anticipation and pain stimulation. Eur J Pain 2006;10(7):659–65.
33. Kaptchuk TJ. Powerful placebo: the dark side of the randomised controlled trial. Lancet 1998;351(9117):1722–5.
34. Hrobjartsson A. What are the main methodological problems in the estimation of placebo effects? J Clin Epidemiol 2002;55(5):430–5.
35. Miller FG, Kaptchuk TJ. The power of context: reconceptualizing the placebo effect. J R Soc Med 2008;101(5):222–5.
36. Moerman DE, Jonas WB. Deconstructing the placebo effect and finding the meaning response. Ann Intern Med 2002;136(6):471–6.
37. Kaptchuk TJ, Kelley JM, Conboy LA, et al. Components of placebo effect: randomised controlled trial in patients with irritable bowel syndrome. BMJ 2008;336(7651):999–1003.
38. Cremonini F, Delgado-Aros S, Camilleri M. Efficacy of alosetron in irritable bowel syndrome: a meta-analysis of randomized controlled trials. Neurogastroenterol Motil 2003;15(1):79–86.
39. Lesbros-Pantoflickova D, Michetti P, Fried M, et al. Meta-analysis: the treatment of irritable bowel syndrome. Aliment Pharmacol Ther 2004;20(11–12):1253–69.
40. Jadad AR, Moore RA, Carroll D, et al. Assessing the quality of reports of randomized clinical trials: is blinding necessary? Control Clin Trials 1996;17(1):1–12.
41. Kirsch I, Moore TJ, Scoboria A, et al. The emperor's new drugs: an analysis of antidepressant medication data submitted to the U.S. Food and Drug Administration. Prev Treat 2002;5. DOI: 10.1037/1522–3736.5.1.523a.
42. Walach H, Maidhof C. Is the placebo effect dependent on time? In: Kirsch I, editor. Expectance, experience, and behavior. Washington, DC: American Psychological Association; 1999. p. 321–32.
43. Walach H, Sadaghiani C, Dehm C, et al. The therapeutic effect of clinical trials: understanding placebo response rates in clinical trials–a secondary analysis. BMC Med Res Methodol 2005;5(26):1–12.
44. Staud R, Price DD. Importance of measuring placebo factors in complex clinical trials. Pain 2008;138:473–4.

45. Staud R, Price DD. Role of placebo factors in clinical trials with special focus on enrichment designs. Pain 2008;139:479–80.
46. Thornton A, Lee P. Publication bias in meta-analysis: its causes and consequences. J Clin Epidemiol 2000;53(2):207–16.
47. Turner EH, Matthews AM, Linardatos E, et al. Selective publication of antidepressant trials and its influence on apparent efficacy. N Engl J Med 2008;358(3): 252–60.
48. McDonald CJ, Mazzuca SA, McCabe GP Jr. How much of the placebo 'effect' is really statistical regression? Stat Med 1983;2(4):417–27.
49. Verhoef MJ, Casebeer AL, Hilsden RJ. Assessing efficacy of complementary medicine: adding qualitative research methods to the "Gold Standard". J Altern Complement Med 2002;8(3):275–81.
50. Ritenbaugh C, Verhoef M, Fleishman S, et al. Whole systems research: a discipline for studying complementary and alternative medicine. Altern Ther Health Med 2003;9(4):32–6.
51. Weatherley-Jones E, Thompson EA, Thomas KJ. The placebo-controlled trial as a test of complementary and alternative medicine: observations from research experience of individualised homeopathic treatment. Homeopathy 2004;93(4):186–9.
52. Institute of Medicine. Need for innovative designs in research on CAM and conventional medicine. Complementary and alternative medicine in the United States. National Academic Press 2005;(4):108–28.
53. Vickers AJ, Rees RW, Zollman CE, et al. Acupuncture of chronic headache disorders in primary care: randomised controlled trial and economic analysis. Health Technol Assess 2004;8(48):iii, 1–35.
54. [ANON]. United Kingdom back pain exercise and manipulation (UK BEAM) randomised trial: cost effectiveness of physical treatments for back pain in primary care. BMJ 2004;329(7479):1381.
55. King M, Nazareth I, Lampe F, et al. Impact of participant and physician intervention preferences on randomized trials: a systematic review. JAMA 2005; 293(9):1089–99.
56. Bower P, King M, Nazareth I, et al. Patient preferences in randomised controlled trials: conceptual framework and implications for research. Soc Sci Med 2005; 61(3):685–95.
57. Johnston BC, Mills E. n-of-1 randomized controlled trials: an opportunity for complementary and alternative medicine evaluation. J Altern Complement Med 2004;10(6):979–84.
58. Hankey GJ. Are n-of-1 trials of any practical value to clinicians and researchers? In: Rothwell PM, editor. The lancet: treating individuals: from randomized trials to personalized medicine. Edinburgh (Scotland): Elsevier Health Sciences; 2007. p. 231–44.

Tai Chi and Rheumatic Diseases

Chenchen Wang, MD, MSc

KEYWORDS

- Tai chi • Mind-body exercise • Osteoarthritis
- Rheumatoid arthritis • Fibromyalgia
- Complementary and alternative medicine • Pain management

Tai chi, a traditional Chinese mind-body exercise, has recently grown in popularity in the United States. According to the 2007 National Health Interview Survey, around 2.5 million Americans have practiced tai chi for health and this number is increasing.[1] Furthermore, individuals with musculoskeletal conditions are more likely to practice tai chi.[2] It is clear that patients with rheumatic disease are interested in seeking this type of complementary and alternative treatment. Thus, it is important to examine evidence-based tai chi mind-body medicine to provide clinicians with an overview of these new sources of knowledge for the best care of rheumatic patients.

As an original Chinese martial art, tai chi has been practiced in China for many centuries. It combines deep diaphragmatic breathing and relaxation with many fundamental postures that flow imperceptibly and smoothly from one to the other through slow, gentle, graceful movements. It has been considered a complex multicomponent intervention integrating physical, psychosocial, emotional, spiritual, and behavioral elements and promoting the mind-body interaction.[3–5] Tai chi evolved into many different styles during its development, including Chen style, Wu style, Sun style, Yang style (classical long form style of 108 postures or simplified style of 24 postures), and other modified styles. Tai chi can be practiced in almost any setting because it requires no equipment and a minimal amount of space.

In the past 2 decades, the potential therapeutic benefits of tai chi for chronic conditions have been consistently recognized in the literature. Significant improvement has

Funding support: This work was supported by the National Center for Complementary and Alternative Medicine of the National Institutes of Health (R21AT003621), the American College of Rheumatology Health Professional Investigator Award, and Boston Claude Pepper Older Americans Independence Center Career Development Award.

Disclaimer: The contents of this article are solely the responsibility of the author and do not necessarily represent the official views of the National Center for Complementary and Alternative Medicine or the National Institutes of Health. The sponsors had no role in the design and conduct of the study; collection, management, analysis, and interpretation of the data; and preparation, review, or approval of the manuscript.

Division of Rheumatology, Tufts Medical Center, Tufts University School of Medicine, 800 Washington Street, Box 406, Boston, MA 02111, USA
E-mail address: cwang2@tuftsmedicalcenter.org

Rheum Dis Clin N Am 37 (2011) 19–32
doi:10.1016/j.rdc.2010.11.002
0889-857X/11/$ – see front matter © 2011 Elsevier Inc. All rights reserved.

been reported in balance, strength, flexibility, cardiovascular and respiratory function, mood, depression and anxiety, self-efficacy, pain reduction, and health-related quality of life in diverse eastern and western populations.[4] Several recent reviews have further suggested that tai chi seems to improve a variety of medical conditions.[6-10]

This article encompasses scientific evidence on the therapeutic benefits of tai chi for several major rheumatic disorders such as osteoarthritis (OA), rheumatoid arthritis (RA), and fibromyalgia (FM). The role of tai chi on associated conditions including neuromuscular abnormalities, cardiovascular disease, osteoporosis, depression, and sleep disturbance is also briefly reviewed.

TAI CHI AND OA

OA, the most prevalent joint disorder, is an increasing problem in the elderly, resulting in chronic pain, functional limitation, reduced quality of life, and substantial health care costs worldwide.[11] The pathophysiological basis of OA is multifaceted and includes impaired muscle function, reduced proprioceptive acuity, and the psychological traits of chronic pain. Symptomatic OA is the most frequent cause of dependency in lower limb tasks, with substantial physical and psychosocial disability.[12-14] Few effective disease-modifying remedies for OA currently exist. Nonsteroidal antiinflammatory drugs (NSAIDs) and acetaminophen, the most widely used therapeutic agents, relieve pain levels by about 20% and carry a hidden cost of serious adverse events in the elderly.[15] Furthermore, recent evidence indicates that arthroscopic surgery for knee OA provides no additional benefits over optimized physical and medical therapy.[16] Recommended core treatments for OA include physical therapy, such as aerobic and muscle strengthening exercises,[17,18] but current data suggest that these treatments have modest benefits for pain and physical function,[19,20] have substantial costs,[21] and may not affect psychological outcomes.[19] In addition, reduced activity levels caused by OA result in poor aerobic capacity and increased risk for cardiovascular disease, obesity, and other inactivity-related conditions.[22-24]

As a complementary mind-body approach, tai chi may be an especially applicable treatment of older adults with OA. The physical component provides exercise consistent with current recommendations for OA (muscle strength, balance, flexibility, and aerobic cardiovascular exercise),[17,18] and the mental component could address the chronic pain state through effects on psychological well-being, life satisfaction, and perceptions of health.[25] These effects may reduce pain, improve function, and retard disease progression and disability associated with OA.[26]

Several randomized controlled studies have examined the effects of tai chi on symptomatic OA. Hartman and colleagues[27] were among the first to conduct a prospective randomized controlled clinical trial to test the efficacy of practicing 12 weeks of tai chi in patients with OA. A total of 35 community-dwelling participants were randomly assigned to receive either two 1-hour tai chi classes per week for 12 weeks (a 9 form Yang style) or to a control group that received usual physical activities and routine care. The results of tai chi training significantly improved arthritis symptoms, arthritis self-efficacy, level of tension, and satisfaction with general health status. In another study, Song and colleagues[28] reported that among 72 patients with OA, patients performing 12 forms of Sun-style tai chi over 12 weeks perceived significantly less pain and stiffness than patients receiving routine treatment. In addition, physical functioning, balance, and abdominal muscle strength were significantly improved in the tai chi group.

In a 3-armed randomized clinical trial of 152 older patients with chronic symptomatic hip and knee OA, Fransen and colleagues[29] found that when compared with a waiting list control group, both 12-week tai chi and hydrotherapy classes provided large and sustained improvements in physical function. All significant improvements were sustained at 24 weeks. In a study by Brismee and colleagues,[30] a 6-week group tai chi program followed by 6 weeks of home tai chi training showed significant improvement in knee pain and physical function compared with an attention control in 41 elderly patients with knee OA; however, the benefits for knee pain (visual analog scale) and the Western Ontario and McMaster Universities (WOMAC) OA overall scores were not sustained throughout the follow-up detraining period (weeks 13–18).

The author's research group has recently conducted a single-blind randomized controlled trial testing the effectiveness of tai chi training in the treatment of knee OA symptoms in the elderly. Forty eligible individuals (aged 55 years or more; with body mass index [calculated as the weight in kilograms divided by height in meters squared] $\leq$40 kg/m^2; with knee pain visual analog scale >40 [range, 0–100]; fulfillment of the American College of Rheumatology [ACR] criteria for knee OA; with radiographic Kellgren and Lawrence grade $\geq$2) were randomly assigned to 60 minutes of tai chi training (10 modified forms from classical Yang style) or an attention control (stretching and wellness education) twice weekly for 12 weeks. The outcomes of the WOMAC OA pain score, WOMAC function, patient and physician global assessments, timed chair stand, depression index, self-efficacy scale, and health-related quality of life were assessed at baseline, 12, 24, and 48 weeks. The results showed that participants in the tai chi arm exhibited significantly greater improvements in pain, physical function, depression, self-efficacy, and health status compared with the controls. Patients who continued tai chi practice after 12 weeks reported durable benefits in pain and function.[31]

Another recent randomized controlled trial of 82 women with OA suggested that 6 months of 31 forms of Sun-style tai chi with qigong breathing exercise significantly improved knee extensor endurance and bone mineral density (BMD) and decreased patients' fear of falling when compared with a self-help education program.[32] Similar positive findings of short- and long-term tai chi have been well documented on balance control, flexibility, muscular strength, and endurance in the elderly,[4,33–36] which have important benefits for patients with symptomatic OA.

Neurologic deficits, especially quadriceps sensory dysfunction (ie, decreased proprioceptive acuity) may precede clinically evident OA and are proposed to be a factor in its pathogenesis and progression. Studies examining the effect of knee joint proprioception and neuromuscular activities have largely focused on older adults with long-term tai chi practice.[37–39] Tsang and Hui-Chan[37] reported a longitudinal study comparing the knee joint proprioception of 21 elderly individuals who practiced tai chi for at least 3 years compared with 21 non–tai chi practicing controls. Using the passive knee joint repositioning test, the tai chi practitioners had better knee joint proprioceptive acuity (less absolute angle errors than controls). This research group further examined knee joint proprioception in 68 elderly subjects who practiced tai chi regularly for at least 4 years, long-term swimming-running exercisers, and sedentary controls. The tai chi practitioners showed significantly better knee joint proprioception than the other 2 groups. In addition, the threshold for detection of passive motion improved in knee flexion and extension in the tai chi group.[38] Moreover, in a cross-sectional study of 61 elderly individuals consisting of long-term tai chi practitioners, regular joggers, and sedentary counterparts, Xu and colleagues[39] found that when compared with a sedentary control, tai chi and jogging groups had significant improvements in the neuromuscular reaction. Despite limited observational evidence, these results generally support that long-term tai chi practice leads to better knee joint proprioceptive acuity and neuromuscular activities in the older population.

In summary, the pathophysiological basis of OA is complex and multifaceted, and symptomatic OA is diverse and heterogeneous. Tai chi exercise, as a multicomponent mind-body intervention, may modulate complex factors and improve health outcomes in OA. The evidence reviewed in this article are promising and suggest that tai chi training may provide an ideal form of exercise for older individuals with OA, suffering from pain and poor function. As a form of physical exercise, tai chi may enhance cardiovascular function, muscular strengthening, proprioceptive acuity, neuromuscular activities, and integration of the mind and body, thereby reducing pain. Stronger muscles and better balance coordination can also improve the stability of joints and physical function. Increased periarticular muscle strength may protect joints from traumatic impacts. Improving self-efficacy, social function, and depression can help people build confidence, get support, and overcome fears of pain, leading to improved physical, psychological, and psychosocial well-being and overall quality of life.[40–42]

TAI CHI AND RA

Treatment of RA, a systemic, diverse, and dynamic disorder, has made major progress over the past few decades. Early active treatment with disease-modifying antirheumatic drugs and biologic agents can be highly beneficial for controlling inflammatory activity and preventing disability in many patients.[43] However, the most effective new drugs can be too expensive and many patients with RA continue to suffer from pain, restricted mobility, reduced muscle strength, and low endurance. In addition, it is increasingly recognized that comorbid conditions play a pivotal role in RA outcomes. For example, cardiovascular complications are the leading contributor to mortality in RA,[44] accounting for approximately one half of all deaths,[45] and osteoporosis resulting in bone fractures represents a major source of morbidity in RA.[46] Indeed, lifestyle behavioral modification is considered to be critical in preventing RA-associated comorbidities and their complications.[47] Tai chi exercise may be beneficial to patients with RA because of its effects on muscle strength, stress reduction, and cardiovascular and bone health, as well as improved health-related quality of life.

One early publication by Kirsteins and colleagues[48] reported on 2 nonrandomized controlled trials of 47 and 28 patients with RA with 10 weeks of tai chi training. Disease activity (joint tenderness, number of swollen joints), time taken to walk 50 ft, handgrip strength and a written functional assessment, and exacerbation of joint symptoms were measured. The studies showed that tai chi seems to be safe for patients with RA and may serve as a suitable weight-bearing exercise with the additional potential advantages of stimulating bone growth and strengthening connective tissue.

A Korean randomized controlled study of 31 patients reported by Lee[49] showed that when compared with a usual care group, 6-week tai chi training significantly improved mood and sleep disturbance. Another Korean randomized controlled trial of 61 patients showed that 50 minutes per week of tai chi training for 12 weeks significantly decreased pain and fatigue compared with usual care controls.[50]

To obtain preliminary data on the effects of tai chi on RA, the author's research group conducted a pilot randomized controlled trial.[51] Twenty patients with functional class I or II RA and mean disease duration of 14.5 years were randomly assigned to tai chi or attention control in twice-weekly sessions for 12 weeks. Patients continued to intake routine medications such as NSAIDS, corticosteroids, and disease-modifying antirheumatic drugs and maintained treatment visits with their primary care physician and rheumatologist throughout the conduct of the study. The ACR20 response criterion, functional capacity, health-related quality of life, and the depression index were assessed. At 12 weeks, 5 of 10 patients (50%) randomized to tai chi achieved an ACR 20% response compared with none (0%) in the control ($P = .03$). Tai chi had greater improvement in the disability index ($P = .01$), vitality subscale of the

36-Item Short Form Health Survey (SF-36) ($P = .01$), and the depression index ($P = .003$). Similar trends to improvement were also observed for disease activity, functional capacity, and health-related quality of life. No adverse events were observed and no patients withdrew from the study, suggesting that tai chi is safe and may be beneficial for functional class I or II RA.

A subsequent study of tai chi in patients with RA by Uhlig and colleagues,[52] however, produced inconsistent results. In a before and after comparison study involving 15 female patients with RA aged 40 to 70 years, participating in an 8-week tai chi training, no improvements were seen in disease activity, muscle strength, flexibility, balance, and health status despite the fact that the study suggested that tai chi was a safe and feasible exercise for RA. The same group of investigators using the similar study design for another 15 patients found that a 12-week tai chi program improved lower limb muscle function and endurance at the end of 12 weeks.[53] A Cochrane review examined the evidence of 4 clinical trials in 206 participants, and only 2 of them exclusively included tai chi from nonrandomized controlled trials by Kirsteins and colleagues.[48] The other 2 trials were using multicomponent programs that include combinations of exercise and tai chi.[54,55] The review suggested that tai chi does not exacerbate symptoms of RA and has statistically significant benefits on lower extremity range of motion for people with RA, with ankle range of motion in particular.[56]

As a chronic disorder characterized by inflammation leading to joint destruction, RA has clinically important comorbidities, including cardiovascular complications and osteoporosis. Numerous studies have evaluated the effects of tai chi on cardiovascular and respiratory function.[57–61] Since 1979, results related to the effect of tai chi on cardiovascular and pulmonary function have been reported in 43 eastern and western publications.[4,8,62] Among them, one study[63] reported that the metabolic intensity of the activity seems insufficient to improve cardiorespiratory fitness in healthy young adults. Yet, other studies suggested that regular tai chi practice may preserve cardiorespiratory function in older individuals and may be prescribed as a suitable exercise for older adults. Recent systematic reviews of the literature have shown that tai chi can reduce blood pressure and increase cardiovascular exercise capacity.[8,62] Thus, encouraging evidence suggests that tai chi may be a safe and beneficial adjunctive therapy to conventional care for patients with RA-associated cardiovascular disease and RA complications. Several large ongoing trials studying tai chi for patients with cardiac conditions will provide more information on the role of tai chi's benefits and mechanisms in the prevention and management of cardiovascular disease.

Evidence from several recent randomized controlled trials and observational studies have evaluated the potential beneficial effects of tai chi for osteoporosis, another common RA-associated comorbidity. In a recent randomized trial comparing 3 times per week tai chi or resistance exercise with a no-intervention control in 180 community-living elders, Woo and colleagues[64] reported that both tai chi and resistance exercise had less BMD loss at total hip after 12 months than the no-intervention controls. In a second randomized trial among 28 sedentary elderly adults, Shen and colleagues[65] compared the effects of tai chi and resistance training and found that treatment with 3 sessions per week of 24-week tai chi increased serum bone-specific alkaline phosphatase and parathyroid hormone levels compared with resistance training after 6 or 12 weeks. Results also revealed a reduction of the urinary calcium level with tai chi at 24 weeks and suggested that tai chi is beneficial for increased bone formation in the elderly. A longitudinal randomized prospective trial also showed that 12 months of 108 form tai chi slowed bone loss in weight-bearing bones in 132 healthy postmenopausal women compared with sedentary controls.[66] Among early postmenopausal Chinese women in Hong Kong, Qin and colleagues[67] demonstrated that tai chi practitioners with more than 4 years experience had significantly higher BMD in the lumbar spine, proximal femur, and distal tibia than sedentary controls. They also demonstrated that regular long-term tai chi practice was associated with higher BMD and better neuromuscular function.[68]

In summary, as a complex immunologically mediated disorder, RA is still a therapeutically challenging chronic condition to control. Emerging evidence from clinical trials reviewed in this article support the concept that the development of better lifestyle-modifying strategies, such as tai chi, could affect the progression of disease and decrease morbidity among individuals with RA. Although existing evidence regarding tai chi on RA remain limited and inconclusive,[69,70] these promising results suggest that tai chi may be a safe adjunctive therapy for RA and warrants further investigation.

TAI CHI AND FM

FM is a complex disorder characterized by widespread musculoskeletal pain, sleep disturbances, functional limitations, and poor quality of life that can be best managed with multidisciplinary therapies.[71,72] Pharmacologic therapies that are currently available for the treatment of FM are associated with numerous limitations, including side effects and addiction and tolerance issues, and patients are often left with unrelieved pain. Nonpharmacologic approaches, including educational and exercise programs, have a role in pain management, but data from clinical trials on the use of these treatment modalities and knowledge of how to best incorporate them into the clinical care of patients are limited.[73]

Recent research testing tai chi mind-body interventions has found considerable benefits for patients with FM. One nonrandomized study of tai chi in 39 individuals with FM suggested that 6 weeks of 1-hour twice-weekly tai chi exercise led to statistically significant improvement in FM symptom management and health-related quality of life.[74] The author's group recently conducted a single-blind randomized controlled trial of classical Yang-style tai chi versus a control intervention consisting of wellness education and stretching for the treatment of FM (defined by the ACR 1990 criteria). Each session lasted 60 minutes and took place twice a week for 12 weeks for each of the study groups. The primary end point was a change in the FM impact questionnaire (FIQ) score (range, 0–100; with higher scores indicating more severe symptoms) at the end of 12 weeks. Secondary end points included patient and physician global assessments, sleep quality, 6-minute walk time, depression, chronic pain, self-efficacy, and summary scores on the physical and mental components of the Medical Outcomes Study SF-36. All assessments were repeated at 24 weeks to test the durability of the response. The study found that when compared with the control group, the 33 patients in the tai chi group had clinically important improvement in the FIQ score and in the measure used to assess pain, sleep quality, depression, and quality of life. Improvements were maintained at 24 weeks. No adverse events were reported in the study participants. Notably, more subjects had discontinued medication use for FM in the tai chi group than in the control group, although the difference was not significant (11 of 31 patients vs 4 of 26, respectively; $P = .09$).[75] Both studies suggested that tai chi may be a useful treatment in the multidisciplinary management of this therapeutically challenging disorder. Similar positive findings were reported in several clinical trials supporting the benefits of other forms of mind-body practice or group exercise, such as qigong, for symptom management in FM.[76–81]

Effect of Tai Chi on Psychological Health

Chronic pain in FM is commonly accompanied by psychosocial stress, anxiety, and depression.[82] Therapeutic approaches with psychological and behavioral effects, such as tai chi mind-body therapy, could better patients' emotional health outcomes.[83]

The author's group systematically reviewed the evidence of the effects of tai chi on stress, anxiety, depression, and mood disturbance in various eastern and western populations.[6] Specifically, the results of 33 randomized and nonrandomized trials suggest that regular tai chi practice is significantly associated with improvements in psychological well-being, including reduced stress (effect size, 0.66; 95% confidence interval [CI], 0.23–1.09), anxiety (effect size, 0.66; 95% CI, 0.29–1.03), depression (effect size, 0.56; 95% CI, 0.31–0.80), and mood disturbance (effect size, 0.45; 95% CI, 0.20–0.69) in healthy participants and patients with chronic conditions (**Fig. 1**). Seven observational studies with relatively large sample sizes reinforced the beneficial association between tai chi practice and psychological health. Notably, the review found that tai chi tends to reduce depression compared with various controls among healthy adults; individuals with OA, RA, FM, depression disorders; sedentary obese women; and elderly participants with cardiovascular disease risk factors. This positive result was associated with improvement in symptoms and physical function in patients with OA, FM, RA, and multiple sclerosis. Interestingly, the benefits were also associated with an improvement in the immune response, with 50% improvement in varicella-zoster virus–specific cell-mediated immunity (T cell–dependent response) after 15 and 25 weeks of tai chi in healthy elderly Americans.[84,85]

However, the vast majority of the studies have less rigorous designs and were conducted on healthy populations, with only 2 studies reporting results on participants diagnosed with clinical depression. Nevertheless, the potential mental health benefits of tai chi mind-body therapy support its inclusion as a key component of a multidisciplinary medical approach to promote psychological health, treat chronic pain, and better inform clinical decision making for FM.

Effect of Tai Chi on Sleep Quality

Sleep disturbances are common in FM, and patients may derive greater benefits from mind-body interventions to improve sleep quality and reduce pain and fatigue. Several randomized controlled studies have investigated the efficacy of tai chi interventions for sleep quality. Li and colleagues[86] randomized 118 older people with moderate sleep disturbance into 1-hour thrice-weekly sessions of tai chi or low-impact exercise for 24 weeks. Tai chi participants reported significant improvements in Pittsburgh Sleep Quality Index global scores and subscores (sleep quality, sleep-onset latency, sleep duration, sleep efficiency, and sleep disturbances) in comparison with the low-impact exercise control group. The study concluded that tai chi seems to be effective as a nonpharmacologic approach for sleep-disturbed elderly individuals. A second randomized controlled trial was reported by Irwin and colleagues[87] on 112 healthy older adults who were randomly assigned to 16 weeks of tai chi training or health education followed by practice and assessment 9 weeks later. The main outcome measure was sleep quality, as assessed by the Pittsburgh Sleep Quality Index. Among adults with moderate sleep disturbance, subjects in the tai chi group showed significant improvements in Pittsburgh Sleep Quality Index global score ($P<.001$), as well as habitual sleep efficiency ($P<.05$), sleep duration ($P<.01$), and sleep disturbance ($P<.01$). In addition, Yeh and colleagues[88] assessed the effects of a 12-week tai chi exercise program on sleep using the sleep spectrogram in a randomized controlled trial of 18 patients with chronic stable heart failure. Compared with the usual care

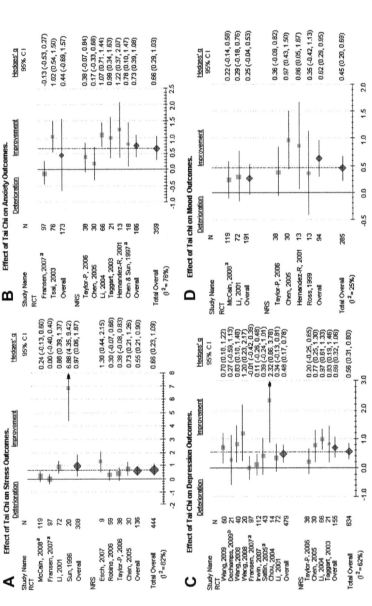

Fig. 1. Effects of tai chi on stress, anxiety, depression, and mood outcomes (*A–D*). The magnitude of the effect size (Hedges' g) (clinical effects) is indicated as 0 to 0.19, negligible effect; 0.20 to 0.49, small effect; 0.50 to 0.79, moderate effect; and 0.80+, large effect. N, number of participants; NRS, nonrandomized comparison study (all the meta-analyzed NRS are self-comparison studies); RCT, randomized controlled trial. [a]McCain 2008, included only tai chi versus waiting list control (n = 119); Fransen 2007, included only tai chi versus control group (n = 97); Chen and Sun 1997, included only participants in tai chi group as pretreatment and posttreatment (n = 18); Sattin 2005, included only clinically depressed participants in tai chi and control arms (n = 43). [b]Dechamps 2009, compared an active control with tai chi. (*Adapted from* Wang C, Bannuru R, Ramel, et al. Tai chi on psychological well-being: systematic review and meta-analysis. BMC Complement Altern Med 2010;10:23. [According to BioMed Central policy, the article permits unrestricted use, distribution, and reproduction in any medium, provided the original work is properly cited.])

group, the tai chi group had significant improvements in sleep stability. Similarly, one observational study of 145 subjects reported that 1 to 14 years of tai chi practice significantly improved sleep and mood disturbance in elderly Chinese participants.[89]

Practicing Tai Chi for Chronic Rheumatic Conditions

Overall, despite limited data, previous works have demonstrated that tai chi, a traditional Chinese mind-body exercise, may be highly suited to the management of symptoms of common chronic rheumatic conditions by reducing pain and improving physical and psychological health and well-being. Scientific research is under way to learn more about how tai chi affects rheumatic diseases and for which conditions it may be helpful. For patients who like to practice tai chi to improve their health and well-being, health care providers need to discuss complementary and alternative practices to help ensure coordinated and safe care. There is no evidence to support that tai chi can be a replacement for conventional care or can postpone visiting a doctor about a medical problem. Also, there is no current standard training for instructors; therefore, providing patients with access to experienced tai chi instructors is essential.

SUMMARY

OA, RA, and FM consist of complex interplay between psychological and biologic aspects. Many patients with these chronic rheumatic illnesses experience high levels of pain and psychological distress that are incompletely relieved by current pharmacologic or physical interventions. Tai chi, a complex multicomponent mind-body therapy, may be particularly applicable for promoting overall quality of life for patients with these chronic rheumatic conditions.

Over the past 2 decades, clinical trials and observational studies have provided encouraging evidence that tai chi, both short- and long-term, has great benefits for patients with a variety of chronic conditions. As a form of physical exercise, tai chi enhances cardiovascular fitness, muscular strength, balance, coordination, and physical function. In addition, tai chi seems to be associated with improvements in psychological well-being including reduced stress, anxiety, depression, and mood disturbance and increased self-esteem. Thus, despite the noted limitations in the evidence, and the need for further methodologically rigorous studies, tai chi mind-body exercise can be safely recommended to patients with OA and FM as a primary form of treatment or as an adjective therapy for RA and its comorbidities to promote both physical and psychological well-being. Further exploring the mechanisms of successful mind-body medicine is important to better inform clinical decision making for rheumatic patients.

ACKNOWLEDGMENTS

The author gratefully acknowledges Dr Robert Kalish and Dr William F. Harvey for their valuable comments and Marcie Griffith's assistance for this review.

REFERENCES

1. Barnes PM, Bloom B, Nahin RL. Complementary and alternative medicine use among adults and children: United States, 2007. Natl Health Stat Report 2009; 12:1–23.
2. Birdee GS, Wayne PM, Davis RB, et al. T'ai chi and qigong for health: patterns of use in the United States. J Altern Complement Med 2009;15:969–73.

3. Yan JH, Downing J. Tai chi. J Aging Phys Activity 1998;6:350–62.
4. Wang C, Collet JP, Lau J. The effect of tai chi on health outcomes in patients with chronic conditions: a systematic review. Arch Intern Med 2004;164:493–501.
5. Wayne PM, Kaptchuk TJ. Challenges inherent to t'ai chi research: part I–t'ai chi as a complex multicomponent intervention. J Altern Complement Med 2008;14:95–102.
6. Wang C, Bannuru R, Ramel J, et al. Tai chi on psychological well-being: systemic review and meta-analysis. BMC Complement Altern Med 2010;10:23.
7. Rogers CE, Larkey LK, Keller C. A review of clinical trials of tai chi and qigong in older adults. West J Nurs Res 2009;31:245–79.
8. Yeh GY, Wang C, Wayne PM, et al. Tai chi exercise for patients with cardiovascular conditions and risk factors: a systematic review. J Cardiopulm Rehabil Prev 2009;29:152–60.
9. Adler PA, Roberts BL. The use of tai chi to improve health in older adults. Orthop Nurs 2006;25:122–6.
10. Jahnke R, Larkey L, Rogers C, et al. A comprehensive review of health benefits of qigong and tai chi. Am J Health Promot 2010;24:e1–25.
11. Felson DT. Clinical practice. Osteoarthritis of the knee. N Engl J Med 2006;354:841–8.
12. van Baar ME, Dekker J, Lemmens JA, et al. Pain and disability in patients with osteoarthritis of hip or knee: the relationship with articular, kinesiological, and psychological characteristics. J Rheumatol 1998;25:125–33.
13. Slemenda C, Brandt KD, Heilman DK, et al. Quadriceps weakness and osteoarthritis of the knee. Ann Intern Med 1997;127:97–104.
14. Rejeski WJ, Miller ME, Foy C, et al. Self-efficacy and the progression of functional limitations and self-reported disability in older adults with knee pain. J Gerontol B Psychol Sci Soc Sci 2001;56:S261–5.
15. Griffin MR, Ray WA, Schaffner W. Nonsteroidal anti-inflammatory drug use and death from peptic ulcer in elderly persons. Ann Intern Med 1988;109:359–63.
16. Kirkley A, Birmingham TB, Litchfield RB, et al. A randomized trial of arthroscopic surgery for osteoarthritis of the knee. N Engl J Med 2008;359:1097–107.
17. Zhang W, Moskowitz RW, Nuki G, et al. OARSI recommendations for the management of hip and knee osteoarthritis, part II: OARSI evidence-based, expert consensus guidelines. Osteoarthr Cartil 2008;16:137–62.
18. Zhang W, Moskowitz RW, Nuki G, et al. OARSI recommendations for the management of hip and knee osteoarthritis, part I: critical appraisal of existing treatment guidelines and systematic review of current research evidence. Osteoarthr Cartil 2007;15:981–1000.
19. Jamtvedt G, Dahm KT, Christie A, et al. Physical therapy interventions for patients with osteoarthritis of the knee: an overview of systematic reviews. Phys Ther 2008;88:123–36.
20. Lange AK, Vanwanseele B, Fiatarone Singh MA. Strength training for treatment of osteoarthritis of the knee: a systematic review. Arthritis Rheum 2008;59:1488–94.
21. Thomas KS, Miller P, Doherty M, et al. Cost effectiveness of a two-year home exercise program for the treatment of knee pain. Arthritis Rheum 2005;53:388–94.
22. Philbin EF, Groff GD, Ries MD, et al. Cardiovascular fitness and health in patients with end-stage osteoarthritis. Arthritis Rheum 1995;38:799–805.
23. Minor MA. Physical activity and management of arthritis. Ann Behav Med 1990;13:385–95.
24. Ries MD, Philbin EF, Groff GD. Relationship between severity of gonarthrosis and cardiovascular fitness. Clin Orthop Relat Res 1995;313:169–76.

25. Axford J, Heron C, Ross F, et al. Management of knee osteoarthritis in primary care: pain and depression are the major obstacles. J Psychosom Res 2008;64:461–7.
26. Sharma L, Cahue S, Song J, et al. Physical functioning over three years in knee osteoarthritis: role of psychosocial, local mechanical, and neuromuscular factors. Arthritis Rheum 2003;48:3359–70.
27. Hartman CA, Manos TM, Winter C, et al. Effects of t'ai chi training on function and quality of life indicators in older adults with osteoarthritis. J Am Geriatr Soc 2000; 48:1553–9.
28. Song R, Lee EO, Lam P, et al. Effects of tai chi exercise on pain, balance, muscle strength, and perceived difficulties in physical functioning in older women with osteoarthritis: a randomized clinical trial. J Rheumatol 2003;30:2039–44.
29. Fransen M, Nairn L, Winstanley J, et al. Physical activity for osteoarthritis management: a randomized controlled clinical trial evaluating hydrotherapy or tai chi classes. Arthritis Rheum 2007;57:407–14.
30. Brismee JM, Paige RL, Chyu MC, et al. Group and home-based tai chi in elderly subjects with knee osteoarthritis: a randomized controlled trial. Clin Rehabil 2007; 21:99–111.
31. Wang C, Schmid CH, Hibberd PL, et al. Tai chi is effective in treating knee osteoarthritis: a randomized controlled trial. Arthritis Rheum 2009;61:1545–53.
32. Song R, Roberts BL, Lee EO, et al. A randomized study of the effects of t'ai chi on muscle strength, bone mineral density, and fear of falling in women with osteoarthritis. J Altern Complement Med 2010;16:227–33.
33. Wayne PM, Krebs DE, Wolf SL, et al. Can tai chi improve vestibulopathic postural control? Arch Phys Med Rehabil 2004;85:142–52.
34. Howe TE, Rochester L, Jackson A, et al. Exercise for improving balance in older people. Cochrane Database Syst Rev 2007;4:CD004963.
35. Sjosten N, Vaapio S, Kivela SL. The effects of fall prevention trials on depressive symptoms and fear of falling among the aged: a systematic review. Aging Ment Health 2008;12:30–46.
36. Low S, Ang LW, Goh KS, et al. A systematic review of the effectiveness of tai chi on fall reduction among the elderly. Arch Gerontol Geriatr 2009;48:325–31.
37. Tsang WW, Hui-Chan CW. Effects of tai chi on joint proprioception and stability limits in elderly subjects. Med Sci Sports Exerc 2003;35:1962–71.
38. Xu D, Hong Y, Li J, et al. Effect of tai chi exercise on proprioception of ankle and knee joints in old people. Br J Sports Med 2004;38:50–4.
39. Xu DQ, Li JX, Hong Y. Effect of regular tai chi and jogging exercise on neuromuscular reaction in older people. Age Ageing 2005;34:439–44.
40. O'Reilly SC, Jones A, Muir KR, et al. Quadriceps weakness in knee osteoarthritis: the effect on pain and disability. Ann Rheum Dis 1998;57:588–94.
41. Backgrounder: tai chi for health purposes. National Center for Complementary and Alternative Medicine, NIH; 2008.
42. Wilson IB, Cleary PD. Linking clinical variables with health-related quality of life. A conceptual model of patient outcomes. JAMA 1995;273:59–65.
43. Klareskog L, Catrina AI, Paget S. Rheumatoid arthritis. Lancet 2009;373:659–72.
44. Symmons DP, Jones MA, Scott DL, et al. Long term mortality outcome in patients with rheumatoid arthritis: early presenters continue to do well. J Rheumatol 1998; 25:1072–7.
45. Reilly PA, Cosh JA, Maddison PJ, et al. Mortality and survival in rheumatoid arthritis: a 25 year prospective study of 100 patients. Ann Rheum Dis 1990;49:363–9.
46. Michel BA, Bloch DA, Fries JF. Predictors of fractures in early rheumatoid arthritis. J Rheumatol 1991;18:804–8.

47. Keefe FJ, Somers TJ, Martire LM. Psychologic interventions and lifestyle modifications for arthritis pain management. Rheum Dis Clin North Am 2008;34:351–68.
48. Kirsteins AE, Dietz F, Hwang SM. Evaluating the safety and potential use of a weight-bearing exercise, Tai-Chi Chuan, for rheumatoid arthritis patients. Am J Phys Med Rehabil 1991;70:136–41.
49. Lee EO. Effects of a tai-chi program on pain, sleep disturbance, mood and fatigue in rheumatoid arthritis patients. Journal of Muscle and Joint Health 2005;12:57–68.
50. Lee KY, Jeong OY. [Effects of a tai-chi program on pain, sleep disturbance, mood and fatigue in rheumatoid arthritis patients]. Taehan Kanho Hakhoe Chi 2006;36:278–85 [in Korean].
51. Wang C. Tai chi improves pain and functional status in adults with rheumatoid arthritis: results of a pilot single-blinded randomized controlled trial. Med Sport Sci 2008;52:218–29.
52. Uhlig T, Larsson C, Hjorth AG, et al. No improvement in a pilot study of tai chi exercise in rheumatoid arthritis. Ann Rheum Dis 2005;64:507–9.
53. Uhlig T, Fongen C, Steen E, et al. Exploring tai chi in rheumatoid arthritis: a quantitative and qualitative study. BMC Musculoskelet Disord 2010;11:43.
54. Van Deusen J, Harlowe D. The efficacy of the ROM Dance Program for adults with rheumatoid arthritis. Am J Occup Ther 1987;41:90–5.
55. Jiang J, Jianyong G, Haiqin Q. A controlled study of San Pi Tang decoction with exercise in the treatment of rheumatoid arthritis. J Integrated Chin Tradit Med West Med 1999;19:588.
56. Han A, Robinson V, Judd M, et al. Tai chi for treating rheumatoid arthritis. Cochrane Database Syst Rev 2004;3:CD004849.
57. Lai JS, Wong MK, Lan C, et al. Cardiorespiratory responses of Tai Chi Chuan practitioners and sedentary subjects during cycle ergometry. J Formos Med Assoc 1993;92:894–9.
58. Lai JS, Lan C, Wong MK, et al. Two-year trends in cardiorespiratory function among older Tai Chi Chuan practitioners and sedentary subjects. J Am Geriatr Soc 1995;43:1222–7.
59. Lan C, Lai JS, Wong MK, et al. Cardiorespiratory function, flexibility, and body composition among geriatric Tai Chi Chuan practitioners. Arch Phys Med Rehabil 1996;77:612–6.
60. Lan C, Lai JS, Wong MK, et al. 12-month tai chi training in the elderly: its effect on health fitness. Med Sci Sports Exerc 1998;30:345–51.
61. Lan C, Chen SY, Lai JS, et al. The effect of tai chi on cardiorespiratory function in patients with coronary artery bypass surgery. Med Sci Sports Exerc 1999;31:634–8.
62. Yeh GY, Wang C, Wayne PM, et al. The effect of tai chi exercise on blood pressure: a systematic review. Prev Cardiol 2008;11:82–9.
63. Zhuo D, Shephard RJ, Plyley MJ, et al. Cardiorespiratory and metabolic responses during Tai Chi Chuan exercise. Can J Appl Sport Sci 1984;9:7–10.
64. Woo J, Hong A, Lau E, et al. A randomised controlled trial of tai chi and resistance exercise on bone health, muscle strength and balance in community-living elderly people. Age Ageing 2007;36:262–8.
65. Shen CL, Williams JS, Chyu MC, et al. Comparison of the effects of tai chi and resistance training on bone metabolism in the elderly: a feasibility study. Am J Chin Med 2007;35:369–81.
66. Chan K, Qin L, Lau M, et al. A randomized, prospective study of the effects of Tai Chi Chun exercise on bone mineral density in postmenopausal women. Arch Phys Med Rehabil 2004;85:717–22.

67. Qin L, Au S, Choy W, et al. Regular Tai Chi Chuan exercise may retard bone loss in postmenopausal women: a case-control study. Arch Phys Med Rehabil 2002; 83:1355–9.

68. Qin L, Choy W, Leung K, et al. Beneficial effects of regular tai chi exercise on musculoskeletal system. J Bone Miner Metab 2005;23:186–90.

69. Lee MS, Pittler MH, Ernst E. Tai chi for rheumatoid arthritis: systematic review. Rheumatology 2007;46:1648–51.

70. Lee MS, Pittler MH, Shin BC, et al. Tai chi for osteoporosis: a systematic review. Osteoporos Int 2008;19:139–46.

71. Wolfe F, Ross K, Anderson J, et al. The prevalence and characteristics of fibromyalgia in the general population. Arthritis Rheum 1995;38:19–28.

72. Goldenberg DL, Burckhardt C, Crofford L. Management of fibromyalgia syndrome. JAMA 2004;292:2388–95.

73. Jones KD, Liptan GL. Exercise interventions in fibromyalgia: clinical applications from the evidence. Rheum Dis Clin North Am 2009;35:373–91.

74. Taggart HM, Arslanian CL, Bae S, et al. Effects of t'ai chi exercise on fibromyalgia symptoms and health-related quality of life. Orthop Nurs 2003;22:353–60.

75. Wang C, Schmid CH, Rones R, et al. A randomized trial of tai chi for fibromyalgia. N Engl J Med 2010;363(8):743–54.

76. Kaplan KH, Goldenberg DL, Galvin-Nadeau M. The impact of a meditation-based stress reduction program on fibromyalgia. Gen Hosp Psychiatry 1993; 15:284–9.

77. Creamer P, Singh BB, Hochberg MC, et al. Sustained improvement produced by nonpharmacologic intervention in fibromyalgia: results of a pilot study. Arthritis Care Res 2000;13:198–204.

78. Astin JA, Berman BM, Bausell B, et al. The efficacy of mindfulness meditation plus qigong movement therapy in the treatment of fibromyalgia: a randomized controlled trial. J Rheumatol 2003;30:2257–62.

79. Sephton SE, Salmon P, Weissbecker I, et al. Mindfulness meditation alleviates depressive symptoms in women with fibromyalgia: results of a randomized clinical trial. Arthritis Rheum 2007;57:77–85.

80. Rooks DS, Gautam S, Romeling M, et al. Group exercise, education, and combination self-management in women with fibromyalgia: a randomized trial. Arch Intern Med 2007;167:2192–200.

81. Lush E, Salmon P, Floyd A, et al. Mindfulness meditation for symptom reduction in fibromyalgia: psychophysiological correlates. J Clin Psychol Med Settings 2009; 16:200–7.

82. Keefe FJ, Bonk V. Psychosocial assessment of pain in patients having rheumatic diseases. Rheum Dis Clin North Am 1999;25:81–103.

83. Bradley LA, Alberts KR. Psychological and behavioral approaches to pain management for patients with rheumatic disease. Rheum Dis Clin North Am 1999;25:215–32.

84. Irwin MR, Pike JL, Cole JC, et al. Effects of a behavioral intervention, Tai Chi Chih, on varicella-zoster virus specific immunity and health functioning in older adults. Psychosom Med 2003;65:824–30.

85. Irwin MR, Olmstead R, Oxman MN. Augmenting immune responses to varicella zoster virus in older adults: a randomized, controlled trial of tai chi. J Am Geriatr Soc 2007;55:511–7.

86. Li F, Fisher KJ, Harmer P, et al. Tai chi and self-rated quality of sleep and daytime sleepiness in older adults: a randomized controlled trial. J Am Geriatr Soc 2004; 52:892–900.

87. Irwin MR, Olmstead R, Motivala SJ. Improving sleep quality in older adults with moderate sleep complaints: a randomized controlled trial of Tai Chi Chih. Sleep 2008;31:1001–8.
88. Yeh GY, Mietus JE, Peng CK, et al. Enhancement of sleep stability with tai chi exercise in chronic heart failure: preliminary findings using an ECG-based spectrogram method. Sleep Med 2008;9:527–36.
89. Long Y, Zang CL, Tang CZ. Effect of Yang style tai chi on sleep, mood for old adults. Occup Health 2000;15:211–2.

Yoga for Arthritis: A Scoping Review

Steffany Haaz, PhD[a],*, Susan J. Bartlett, PhD[b,c]

KEYWORDS

- Yoga • Rheumatoid arthritis • Osteoarthritis • Physical activity
- Exercise • Mindfulness

Yoga includes a variety of theories and practices that originated in ancient India and have evolved and spread throughout the world. In Sanskrit, yoga means "to yoke" or connect.[1] This term typically refers to mind-body integration, but over the thousands of years that yoga has evolved, this focus has also been applied to spatial surroundings, nature, other individuals, and spiritual interconnectedness.[2] The physical practice of yoga, referred to as "hatha," was originally intended to prepare for meditation, an important spiritual practice in many cultures. In recent decades, hatha yoga has become popular for physical activity and stress management. Other aspects of yoga, including study of ancient texts, dietary practices, acts of service, and moral living, may be mentioned but are not generally a focus of western classes.

After attention to posture, deep breathing, and/or chanting, yoga practice often begins with a slow movement sequence to increase blood flow and warm muscles. This sequence is followed by poses that include flexion, extension, adduction, abduction, and rotation.[1,3] Holding poses builds strength by engaging muscles in isometric contraction.[4,5] Moving joints through their full range of motion increases flexibility,[6,7] whereas standing poses promote balance by strengthening and stabilizing muscles and improving proprioception to reduce falls.[8,9] Thus, yoga incorporates several elements of exercise that may be beneficial for arthritis.

To cope with pain, patients with arthritis often reduce activity.[10,11] However, inactivity can result in muscle or tendon shortening, articular capsule contraction, and weakened ligaments.[12] Conversely, regular activity may decrease pain and preserve stability.[12,13]

This work was supported by grant No. F31 AT003362-01A1 from the National Institutes of Health and a Doctoral Dissertation Award from the Arthritis Foundation.
The authors have nothing to disclose.
[a] Department of Health, Behavior and Society, Johns Hopkins School of Public Health, 615 North Wolfe Street, Baltimore, MD 21205, USA
[b] Department of Medicine, McGill University, Montreal, Ontario, H3A 1A1 Canada
[c] Johns Hopkins Division of Rheumatology, 5200 Eastern Avenue, Mason F. Lord, Center Tower, 4th Floor, Baltimore, MD 21224, USA
* Corresponding author. Johns Hopkins Arthritis Center, 5200 Eastern Avenue, Mason F. Lord, Center Tower, 4th Floor, Baltimore, MD 21224.
E-mail address: info@drhaaz.com

Although there was once a concern that exercise might increase inflammation and exacerbate pain, regular physical activity is now recommended as part of the comprehensive treatment of arthritis.[14–17] The American College of Rheumatology (ACR),[18] Osteoarthritis Research Society International (OARSI),[19] and the Ottawa Panel[20] note that stretching, strengthening, and conditioning exercises can preserve physical function, increase strength, and improve endurance for people with arthritis. All persons with arthritis should consult with their doctor to determine a safe and appropriate approach to increasing physical activity.

Unfortunately, long-term exercise maintenance is uncommon even for healthy individuals, generally approaching 50% after 6 months.[21] Vigorous exercise is ideal for physical health[22] and may be acceptable for some persons with arthritis[23,24] but it could be intolerable and may not be recommended for those with significant joint instability or damage.[25,26] Adherence to moderate-intensity exercise is more broadly tolerable but still not attained by most people with arthritis.[27] For patients with arthritis, emphasis on stretching, strength, posture, balance, and the ability to adjust pace and intensity are important components of a safe activity, all of which yoga encompasses. Yoga is multifaceted, including focused breathing, mental engagement, stress management, social connection, and/or meditative concentration, along with physical activity. Yoga may offer an alternative to traditional exercise and potential psychological benefits or increased enjoyment for enhanced exercise adherence. Yoga could, therefore, provide another way for patients with arthritis to be active and engaged in an health-promoting behavior. Mind-body interventions, such as yoga, that teach stress management with physical activity may affect diseases from multiple fronts and may be well suited for investigation in both osteoarthritis (OA) and inflammatory immune-mediated diseases such as rheumatoid arthritis (RA).

The goal of this review is to evaluate existing evidence regarding the effects of yoga practice on clinical, functional, and psychosocial outcomes for people with arthritis.

METHODS

Databases including MEDLINE, PsychLIT, PsychINFO, and IndMed (an Indian database) were searched for research trials published from 1980 through May 2010, using yoga (including poses, breathing practices, relaxation, and/or meditation) as an exercise intervention for patients with arthritis. Additional relevant publications found in references from the original search list are also reviewed. Research in progress was searched via abstracts from annual scientific meetings of the American Public Health Association, ACR, OARSI, European League Against Rheumatism, and International Association of Yoga Therapists. The following search terms were used: yoga or yogic and arthritis, arthritic, rheumatoid, rheumatic, or osteoarthritis. This review is limited to studies including quantitative statistical analysis and peer review.

RESULTS

A total of 11 articles that described evaluating the effects of a yoga intervention in persons with arthritis were examined. One case series was excluded for lack of quantitative methods.[28] Final analysis consisted of 10 studies (**Table 1**). Among the 10 studies, 6 focused on RA, 2 were for OA only, and 2 included both RA and OA or arthritis in general. The studies were all published from 1980 to 2010.

Study Quality

Study quality was assessed based on study design, sample size, intervention protocol, and statistical analysis. Studies were classified as low, moderate, or high.

Table 1
Studies included in systematic review

Authors	Design	Date Published	Participants	Sample Size	Location	Intervention
Article						
Kolasinski et al[39]	Cohort	2005	Knee OA in at least 1 knee, 6/7 obese, aged >50 y, all female	7	Philadelphia, PA, USA	90 min, 1/wk for 8 wk (Iyengar)
Garfinkel et al[30]	RCT, waiting-list control	1994	Hand OA, age 52–79 y, male and female	17	Philadelphia, PA, USA	60 min, 1/wk for 8 wk (Iyengar)
Dash and Telles[34]	Matched controls for age and sex	2001	RA, age 21–43 y, male and female	40	—	15 continuous days
Bosch et al[37]	Convenience control	2009	RA, postmenopausal women	16	—	90 min, 3/wk for 10 wk
Badsha et al[36]	Convenience control	2009	Middle-aged adults with RA, mostly of Indian and Caucasian decent	47	Dubai, UAE	60 min, 2/wk for 6 wk (Raj)
Letter to the editor						
Haslock et al[33]	RCT, usual care control	1994	RA, age 15–72 y	20	Britain	120 min, 5/wk for 3wk; 1/wk for 3 mo; 10–30 min daily home practice
Evans et al[38]	Cohort	2010	RA, young adults	5	Los Angeles, CA, USA	90 min, 2/wk for 6 wk
Abstracts						
Haaz et al[31]	RCT, waiting-list control	2007	RA or knee OA, age 18–65 y, mostly female, mixed racial background	37	Baltimore, MD, USA	60 min, 3/wk for 8 wk; 1/wk home practice
Haaz[32]	RCT, waiting-list control	2008	RA, age 18–65 y, mostly female, mixed racial background	30	Baltimore, MD, USA	60 min, 3/wk for 8 wk; 1/wk home practice
Sharma[35]	Matched controls for age and sex	2005	Any arthritis diagnosis, age 45–66 y, mostly women, all Caucasian	24	Midwestern state, USA	75 min, 1/wk for 6 wk (Kundalini)

Abbreviation: RCT, randomized controlled trial.

These criteria are based on categories set forth by the US Department of Health and Human Services 2002 report.[29] Funding source was not included as a category because most studies did not report a funding source, although the available information about funding was described. Because this review includes both randomized and observational trials, categories were adapted for both (**Table 2**).

Study Design

Of the 10 studies included in this review, 4 were randomized controlled trials (RCTs)[30–33]; 2 compared people with arthritis to healthy controls, matching for age and sex[34,35]; 2 were non-RCTs (NRCTs)[36,37]; and 2 were cohort studies.[38,39] Among the 4 RCTs, 3 had a waiting-list control and the other 2 were usual care. The NRCTs assigned participants to control if they were unable to attend the first class session. None of the studies had an active control group. Of the reviewed studies, 6 were reported as journal articles,[30,34,36–39] 1 was a letter to the editor,[33] and 3 were presented as abstracts at annual research meetings.[31,32] One study was presented as an abstract at an annual meeting, followed by publication in a journal that did not include a process of peer review[35]; therefore, only the abstract was included in this review.

Sample Size

Sample sizes ranged from 3[28] to 26[36] intervention completers, with similar numbers of comparator groups. Only 1 study had as many as 20 persons per group.[36] The necessary sample size to detect differences between groups was not generally described. Generally, a subject to variable item ratio of 10 to 1 is recommended in multivariable regression analysis to avoid type I errors,[40,41] although this ratio depends on variable distribution.[42,43]

Table 2
Study quality scoring based on Health and Human Services recommendations

	Study Quality Score		
	0	1	2
Study Design	Uncontrolled	Matched or convenience control, such as comparing preexisting groups	Randomized controlled trial
Sample Size (Final Data Set)	0–10/group	11–20/group	>20/group
Intervention	Lacking detailed description about the intervention's components and protocol	Comprehensive yoga program with mention of several components (ie, poses, breathing, meditation)	Well-described comprehensive program, including specific poses and/or modifications, images, class structure
Data Analysis	Justification for outcome measures not described or not validated, unnecessary potential for bias, statistical methods not appropriate for the data	Some limitations in collection and analysis of data that are generally recognized and explained by study authors	Hypothesis-driven outcomes; reliable and validated measures, with efforts to reduce measurement bias; and explanation for use of appropriate statistical methods

There were 6 studies reported on attrition, with rates of 0%,[36] 9%,[33] 22%,[30] 36%,[39] and 37% each,[35,38] with the 3 most rigorous studies having the lowest rates of attrition. The 2 cohort trials and 1 trial with healthy matched controls had the highest rates of attrition. The greatest retention was from the NRCTs and 2 RCTs. Most studies analyzed data for completers only. Only 1 study reported the consideration of attrition in final analysis, excluding 1 dropout before baseline.[33] Remaining studies did not report attrition.[31,32,34,44]

Intervention Protocol

Intervention protocols varied widely. The "dose" of yoga varied substantially between studies and was often inconsistent within studies. For example, the study with the greatest dose included 120 minutes of practice 5 times per week followed by once per week for 3 months with 10 to 30 minutes of daily home practice. In contrast, the lowest dose included 60 minutes once per week for 8 weeks. Yet another study was only 15 days long but included daily practice in a retreat setting. Some studies required daily home practice, some weekly, and some had no element of home practice. Although many protocols were developed and/or taught by licensed or certified yoga professionals (teachers, therapists, or scholars), some did not describe the intervention development or delivery. This is further complicated because requirements and regulation of yoga instruction differ by jurisdiction and culture, and credentials of the yoga professionals are not always standardized. Some studies used a style of yoga with a long history and published texts describing teaching methods and practice, whereas others developed a new protocol for the population under investigation. Some studies failed to describe the protocol in any detail.

Three studies, an RCT for hand OA,[30] a cohort study for knee OA,[39] and an NRCT of young adults with RA,[38] used an Iyengar-based yoga program. This style is known for using props (blocks, straps, bolsters) adjusting to individual anatomy.[1] The program for both the OA studies was developed by one of the authors who is a senior certified yoga instructor, and the RA protocol was devised by an experienced Iyengar yoga (IY) teacher.[38] The hand OA trial included 10 weeks of "stretching and strengthening exercises emphasizing extension and alignment, group discussion, supportive encouragement and general questions and answers."[30] Poses emphasized respiration and upper body alignment. The protocol is described generally with reference to a previous publication. The knee OA study described a 15-pose series and prop modifications, which could be easily replicated. The RA study by Evans and colleagues[38] listed examples of poses. The IY-based programs were conducted for 6,[39] 8,[30] and 10[30] weeks, meeting once or twice weekly for 60 to 90 minutes.

An NRCT for RA used a program developed in consultation with rheumatologists and a certified yoga therapist. This program, conducted by Badsha and colleagues,[36] included stretches, strengthening, meditation, and deep breathing of biweekly classes for 6 weeks. A study with healthy matched control by Dash and Telles[34] included poses, breathing practices, meditation, lectures, and joint loosening exercises in a 14-day yoga training camp. The RCT by Haslock and colleagues[33] used gentle tailored poses, breath control, meditation, lectures, and discussions, with the intention to soften emotions. For the first 3 weeks, 120-minute sessions were held 5 days per week, followed by weekly 120-minute sessions for 3 months.

Abstracts from an RCT of RA and OA discussed the use of a gentle yoga program developed by rheumatologists, psychologists, and a registered yoga therapist,[31,32] incorporating poses, breathing practices, relaxation, meditation, chanting, and supplemental reading. A study with age- and sex-matched controls taught a social cognitive theory–based Kundalini yoga intervention to those diagnosed with arthritis.[35] Kundalini yoga concentrates on the spine, with a focus on raising energy and awareness.[45] The study included poses, breathing techniques, meditation, and relaxation. In 2 studies,[33,39] the reader is referred elsewhere for description of the practice.

Data Collection and Analysis

Well-validated instruments were administered by blinded assessors in 6 studies.[28,30,33,34,39,44] These included anatomic changes, biomarkers, performance outcomes, and clinical assessment. The inclusion of unmasked assessors in one study was found to be its greatest limitation.[36]

All but 2 studies[33,35] measured baseline variables and outcomes recommended by ACR or OARSI.[46,47] None used sham yoga to blind participants. Consequently, all self-report data sustain possible expectation bias. However, the chosen self-report instruments are commonly used for persons with arthritis and known for strong psychometric properties.

One study with healthy controls created a new assessment tool to measure intervention efficacy and participant perceptions.[35] The investigators had previously used some of the questions in this population and demonstrated strong validity and reliability. Additions to the tool were checked for face and content validity by 3 academics.

Only 2 trials (an NRCT and a cohort study) reported efforts to ensure that data characteristics supported the methods (such as assuming a normal distribution) and adjusted the statistical plan as necessary.[36,39] Eight articles and abstracts described hypotheses up front and linked outcomes to those hypotheses. The other 2 listed feasibility as their primary outcome.[33,35] However, some outcomes were not well explained in the study's context. For example, a study comparing patients with RA to healthy controls hypothesized that yoga would result in increased strength.[34] However, this study measured pre- and postintervention nonsteroidal antiinflammatory drug (NSAID) dose, without assessing analgesic or other medication use and included no pain measures.

Overall Study Quality

Of 8 possible points, studies ranged from 3 to 6 in overall study quality (**Table 3**). Future expansion from pilot studies and abstracts may include greater rigor. Although available information is limited, the strongest studies can point toward associations that may be confirmed with additional trials.

Table 3
Outcome of study quality assessment, based on criteria in Table 2

Authors	Study Design	Sample Size	Intervention	Data Collection/ Analysis	Overall
Kolasinski et al,[39] 2005	0	0	2	2	4
Garfinkel et al,[30] 1994	2	1	2	1	6
Haslock et al,[33] 1994	2	1	2	1	6
Dash and Telles,[34] 2001	1	1	1	1	4
Sharma,[35] 2005	0	1	1	1	3
Badsha et al,[36] 2009	1	2	2	1	6
Haaz et al,[31] 2007 and Haaz et al,[32] 2008	2	1	1	1	5
Bosch et al,[44] 2003	2	0	1	1	4
Evans et al,[38] 2010	0	0	1	1	2

STUDY FINDINGS

Professional organizations have provided evidence-based recommendations for the use of particular outcomes for RA and OA. ACR suggests that trials of RA use the following measurement tools: tender joint count, swollen joint count, patient pain assessment, patient and physician global assessment of disease activity, patient assessment of physical function, and laboratory evaluation of one acute phase reactant.[46] For OA, OARSI recommends pain as the primary outcome, along with physical function and a patient global assessment.[47] These outcomes can be measured with any tool that has adequate validity, reliability, and responsiveness. Later addition of other outcomes were not ruled out, such as physician global assessment, health-related quality of life (HRQL), inflammation, stiffness, and time to surgery. Although no study included all of the recommended outcomes, most included one or more. See **Table 4** for study findings.

Clinical Outcomes

The Disease Activity Score (DAS) is an index developed to measure RA disease activity that has been extensively validated for use in clinical trials.[48,49] This index includes the number of tender and swollen joints along with the erythrocyte sedimentation rate or C-reactive protein levels and a patient assessment of disease activity. Two RA studies measured DAS-28 (includes a 28 joint count), and both found statistically significant improvements for patients participating in the yoga intervention as compared with controls.[32,36]

Two studies measured ring size as a marker of hand inflammation. Haslock and Ellis[33] reported a trend toward statistical difference in ring size for persons with RA, whereas Garfinkel and colleagues[30] observed no change in ring size in persons with hand OA. A difference in antiinflammatory medications for persons with RA could not be attributed to the intervention because the 2 groups differed at baseline.[34]

Only 1 knee OA study reported on stiffness but found no improvement,[39] although a trend toward improvement for global patient assessment was reported. The hand OA trial saw improved finger tenderness and finger range of motion.[50] A study of general arthritis (diagnostic inclusion criteria unclear) used its own symptom self-report instrument, with no improvements demonstrated.[35]

Functional Ability

Several studies assessed strength, balance, flexibility, and/or mobility. Three studies used hand grip, which has been considered a clinical measure of general strength,[51] hand function, pain, disease activity,[52] and future disability.[53] Improvements were found for 2 RA studies[33,34] but not in the study on hand OA.[30] An NRCT of postmenopausal women with RA showed improved balance,[37] whereas the knee OA pilot study found no change in 50 ft time.[39]

Of the 5 studies in RA, 4 used the Health Assessment Questionnaire (HAQ), a self-report of disability status, as an outcome measure. Two studies found significant improvement compared with controls or baseline,[36,37] and another study showed a trend toward improvement.[33] The HAQ also includes a visual analog scale (VAS) of pain, which was used in 3 of the RA studies. Two studies demonstrated significant improvement,[37,38] whereas 1 study found no change.[36] Although the HAQ is often considered to be a disease-specific tool intended for use in RA, it has also been used more broadly and was included in a study on hand OA.[30] In this study, there was no change in the functional dimension of the HAQ, but pain measured by VAS

Table 4
Study findings

Authors	Study Quality	Clinical Outcomes	Functional Outcomes	Psychosocial Outcomes
Kolasinski et al[39]	4	Improved: WOMAC pain, function Trend: GA No change: stiffness	No change: 15 m walk time	Improved: affect
Garfinkel et al[30]	6	Improved: finger tenderness, hand pain, ROM No change: hand function, ring size	No change: grip strength	—
Haslock et al[33]	6	Trend: HAQ-DI, ring size	Improved: grip strength	No change: GHQ
Dash and Telles[34]	4	—	Improved: grip strength	—
Sharma[35]	3	—	—	Improved: self-efficacy for yoga
Badsha et al[36]	6	Improved: HAQ-DI, DAS-28 No change: HAQ pain	—	No change: physical/mental quality of life
Haaz et al[32]	5	Improved: tender/swollen joints	—	Improved: physical & emotional roles, energy (RA), pain (RA) Trend: mental health, energy (OA), pain (OA)
Bosch et al[44]	4	Improved: HAQ-DI and pain	Improved: balance	Improved: depressive symptoms, daytime cortisol levels Trend: diurnal and awakening cortisol levels
Evans et al[38]	2	Improved: pain (PDI, HAQ) Trend: physical functioning No change: HAQ-DI	—	Improved: vitality, mental health, global severity, self-efficacy Trend: chronic pain acceptance, mindfulness

Abbreviations: DAS-28, Disease Activity Score (includes a 28 joint count); GA, Global Assessment; GHQ, General Health Questionnaire; HAQ-DI, Health Assessment Questionnaire-Disability Index; PDI, Pain Disability Index; ROM, range of motion; WOMAC, Western Ontario and McMaster Osteoarthritis Index.

did improve significantly; however, the HAQ is not as sensitive to changes in persons with OA.[50]

Psychosocial Outcomes

The Arthritis Impact Measurement Scale 2 (AIMS2) and the Medical Outcomes Study 36-Item Short Form Health Survey (SF-36) assess HRQL. The SF-36 is a general measure,[54] whereas the AIMS2 is specifically designed for arthritic patients.[55] Both the measures contain mental and physical domains. The AIMS2 addresses unique issues of this population, but the SF-36 allows for comparison with nonarthritic participants.

Significant improvement in AIMS2 score was seen for knee OA, with a trend toward improved symptoms and patient global assessment. Using the SF-36, one study found no improvements,[36] whereas an abstract reported improved emotional roles and energy, with a trend toward improved mental health.[31]

Improvements in psychosocial health were tracked using other instruments, including the Beck Depression Index.[37] Two RA studies noted no changes in psychological health, measured by the General Health Questionnaire[33] and SF-36.[36] Change in cortisol levels, a common biomarker of psychological stress, was also measured, with significant improvement in daytime measurements and a trend for improved diurnal and awakening levels.[37] Measures of pain included the Western Ontario and McMaster Osteoarthritis Index (WOMAC), a validated index for OA of the knee and hip, for a study of OA[39] and the Pain Disability Index for a study of RA.[37] Improvements in pain were statistically significant in both the studies.[38] Persons with arthritis who practiced Kundalini yoga reported increased self-efficacy and frequency of yoga behaviors.[35]

Medication Use

Two studies required that no changes were made to treatment during the trial,[33,39] and one RA study required stable dose of disease-modifying antirheumatic drugs and a limit to glucocorticoid use.[37] Badsha and colleagues[36] reported reductions in medication use for 3 persons with RA in the yoga group (3 corticosteroids, 1 etanercept, 2 methotrexate) because of clinical improvement and none in the control group. Dash and Telles[34] noted a statistically significant reduction in NSAID use for the intervention group with RA, although groups differed at baseline. Other studies did not report changes in medication or procedures to maintain stable medication use.

Funding Sources

Most articles and abstracts did not disclose whether the study was funded. The study by Badsha and colleagues[36] was funded by the Emirates Arthritis Foundation and by an unrestricted grant from Abbott Pharmaceuticals, with no reported conflicts of interest. Research by Kolasinski and colleagues[39] was partially supported by ACR Clinical Summer Preceptorship Program. The letter to the editor by Haslock and Ellis[33] notes in acknowledgments that "Marks and Spencer contributed to the cost of data processing." No other mention is made of funding support.

DISCUSSION

The assessment of yoga for arthritis is in its infancy. In general, the studies that are reported in the literature are very small in both size and scope. The use of recommended outcomes and validated measures was typical, but only a few outcomes were included in each study. Therefore, there is too little overlap in disease state and measured variables to pool data or draw preliminary conclusions.

HRQL is an important self-reported outcome that can inform about the broad effects of interventions on several life domains. Few studies included HRQL, and none used it as a primary outcome. Although tools like the HAQ and WOMAC measure arthritis disability and its impact on daily activities, they do not assess the 8 domains of health ranging from physical limitations to energy and mental health. In addition, because these tools are primarily used in arthritic populations, comparison with healthy adults or other chronic conditions is not possible.

Study designs varied and each had drawbacks, including lack of masking, lack of control groups, group crossover, and biased group assignment. In these cases, limitations were often noted, but efforts made to reduce bias were not always explained. No study included comparison treatment arms. This exclusion would strengthen findings but requires a larger sample size and greater resources, which is a challenge in time-intensive behavioral research trials.[30]

Yoga describes a range of practices. Although most studies described a comprehensive intervention (poses, breathing, relaxation, and/or meditation), the styles, doses, and format varied. Researchers must be clear about the delivered intervention and that it is population appropriate. Determining which aspects of the practice are safe and beneficial can only follow when it is known what has been tested. Especially, with patients who have considerable musculoskeletal limitations and symptoms, what is taught and how it is modified should be detailed in future research and practice. Beyond this, researchers should provide protocol transparency so that larger more rigorous trials can replicate the interventions using the same methods to confirm or dispute findings. Furthermore, when design methods and statistical analyses are not well described, research cannot be properly evaluated and readers are unable to determine whether methodological flaws may be responsible for errors in findings.

For classroom-based interventions, it may be challenging to recruit participants willing to travel and dedicate several hours per week for months, especially with unpredictable painful diseases. Understudied interventions are often limited to the safest and healthiest people (by age and/or disease status) to ensure no harm before expanding the study to vulnerable populations. Although this practice reduces qualifying participants, particularly for a rarer disease (such as RA), it can bias the sample and limit generalizability to all persons with the disease.

Arthritis encompasses many diagnoses. The 2 most common OA and RA have significant pathophysiologic differences, and effects of an intervention such as yoga may not be the same for each. Moreover, the effects of yoga on isolated hand OA versus knee OA may also have significantly different outcomes. Combining persons with different diseases in the same intervention and analyzing the data collectively could mask an effect that is strong for just a portion of participants or could suggest a universal effect that only applies to a subgroup with one particular form of arthritis. The use of biomarkers as treatment outcomes improves the current understanding of how additional biochemical and pathophysiologic parameters of diseases respond to interventions.

The research in this review was conducted in diverse populations across the globe, which suggests broad interest as well as cross-cultural acceptance. However, perceptions of yoga, teaching methods, and differences in arthritis treatment are likely to influence intervention effects and, possibly, result in different findings.

Overall, the most consistent findings were for tender or swollen joints in persons with RA, which improved for all 3 studies that used this outcome. Another common outcome was pain, which improved in 6 out of 8 studies, measured by various tools.

Disability improved in 3 out of 4 studies. Self-efficacy improved in both studies in which it was measured. Mental health and energy improved in 2 out of 3 studies. For grip strength, improvements were seen in both studies of RA but not in the study of OA that included it. Results for global health and physical functioning were inconsistent. Measures of disease symptoms and physical functioning were more commonly used than markers of physical fitness or psychosocial functioning. Because different instruments were often used to assess the same outcome, interpretation of results across studies is compromised.

A goal of future studies should be to create standardized protocols that are optimized to enhance safety, enjoyment, and long-term adherence (including specific poses and modifications). Studies have varied considerably with regard to the frequency and duration of yoga practice, as well as the style and specific class content. The practice studied should be thoroughly described, including specifying the yoga lineage (Iyengar, Kundalini, and other types) in the Methods section or separately publishing intervention details.

Interdisciplinary collaboration in the design of yoga interventions is appropriate for this population. Yoga experts, rheumatology clinicians, or clinical researchers are not equipped to create an authentic and appropriate yoga program alone without consultation with each other. Such a program requires careful attention to the stress on joints and connective tissue, as well as the consideration of joint range of motion and adaptation during potential disease flares. An arthritis-appropriate program that has been created in careful collaboration and well tested through rigorous research methods is required as a next step in the evolution of this research.

Of significant interest is to study the mechanisms by which yoga affects arthritis symptoms. The use of standardized outcome measures and appropriate statistical methods is essential for confirming findings. Large comprehensive trials are required to validate improvements indicated by this collection of small pilot studies.

REFERENCES

1. Garfinkel M, Schumacher HR Jr. Yoga. Rheum Dis Clin North Am 2000;26(1):125–32, x.
2. McCall T. Yoga as medicine: the yogic prescription for health and healing. New York: Bantam Dell; 2007.
3. Fishman L, Saltonstall E. Yoga for arthritis. New York: W.W. Norton & Company, Inc; 2008.
4. Madanmohan, Thombre DP, Balakumar B, et al. Effect of yoga training on reaction time, respiratory endurance and muscle strength. Indian J Physiol Pharmacol 1992;36(4):229–33.
5. Madanmohan, Mahadevan SK, Balakrishnan S, et al. Effect of six weeks yoga training on weight loss following step test, respiratory pressures, handgrip strength and handgrip endurance in young healthy subjects. Indian J Physiol Pharmacol 2008;52(2):164–70.
6. Tekur P, Singphow C, Nagendra HR, et al. Effect of short-term intensive yoga program on pain, functional disability and spinal flexibility in chronic low back pain: a randomized control study. J Altern Complement Med 2008;14(6):637–44.
7. Oken BS, Kishiyama S, Zajdel D, et al. Randomized controlled trial of yoga and exercise in multiple sclerosis. Neurology 2004;62(11):2058–64.

8. Gauchard GC, Jeandel C, Tessier A, et al. Beneficial effect of proprioceptive physical activities on balance control in elderly human subjects. Neurosci Lett 1999;273(2):81–4.

9. Hart CE, Tracy BL. Yoga as steadiness training: effects on motor variability in young adults. J Strength Cond Res 2008;22(5):1659–69.

10. Bolen J, Murphy L, Greenlund K, et al. Arthritis as a potential barrier to physical activity among adults with heart disease – United States, 2005 and 2007 [report]. MMWR Morb Mortal Wkly Rep 2009;58(7):165–9.

11. Kaplan MS, Huguet N, Newsom JT, et al. Characteristics of physically inactive older adults with arthritis: results of a population-based study. Prev Med 2003; 37(1):61–7.

12. Rheumatoid arthritis: clinical and laboratory features. In: Klippel JH, Crofford LJ, Stone JH, et al, editors. Primer on the rheumatic diseases. Atlanta (GA): Arthritis Foundation; 2001. p. 218–24.

13. de Jong Z, Munneke M, Zwinderman AH, et al. Long term high intensity exercise and damage of small joints in rheumatoid arthritis. Ann Rheum Dis 2004;63(11): 1399–405.

14. Stenstrom CH, Minor MA. Evidence for the benefit of aerobic and strengthening exercise in rheumatoid arthritis. Arthritis Rheum 2003;49(3):428–34.

15. Van den Ende CH, Vliet Vlieland TP, Munneke M, et al. Dynamic exercise therapy in rheumatoid arthritis: a systematic review. Br J Rheumatol 1998; 37(6):677–87.

16. Creamer P, Hochberg MC. Osteoarthritis. Lancet 1997;350(9076):503–8.

17. Blumstein H, Gorevic PD. Rheumatologic illnesses: treatment strategies for older adults. Geriatrics 2005;60(6):28–35.

18. American College of Rheumatology Subcommittee on Rheumatoid Arthritis Guidelines. Guidelines for the management of rheumatoid arthritis: 2002 update. Arthritis Rheum 2002;46(2):328–46.

19. Zhang W, Moskowitz RW, Nuki G, et al. OARSI recommendations for the management of hip and knee osteoarthritis. Part II: OARSI evidence-based, expert consensus guidelines. Osteoarthritis Cartilage 2008;16(2):137–62.

20. Ottawa Panel. Ottawa Panel evidence-based clinical practice guidelines for therapeutic exercises in the management of rheumatoid arthritis in adults. Phys Ther 2004;84(10):934–72.

21. Dishman RK. Compliance/adherence in health-related exercise. Health Psychology 1982;1:1237–67.

22. Pate RR, Pratt M, Blair SN, et al. Physical activity and public health. A recommendation from the centers for disease control and prevention and the American College of Sports Medicine. JAMA 1995;273(5):402–7.

23. Lemmey AB, Marcora SM, Chester K, et al. Effects of high-intensity resistance training in patients with rheumatoid arthritis: a randomized controlled trial. Arthritis Rheum 2009;61(12):1726–34.

24. Bosomworth NJ. Exercise and knee osteoarthritis: benefit or hazard? Can Fam Physician 2009;55(9):871–8.

25. Buckwalter JA, Lane NE. Athletics and osteoarthritis. Am J Sports Med 1997; 25(6):873–81.

26. Minor MA, Lane NE. Recreational exercise in arthritis. Rheum Dis Clin North Am 1996;22(3):563–77.

27. Farr JN, Going SB, Lohman TG, et al. Physical activity levels in patients with early knee osteoarthritis measured by accelerometry. Arthritis Rheum 2008;59(9): 1229–36.

28. Bukowski EL, Conway A, Glentz LA, et al. The effect of Iyengar yoga and strengthening exercises for people living with osteoarthritis of the knee: a case series. Int Q Community Health Educ 2007;26(3):287–305.
29. Scott HS. Systems to rate the strength of scientific evidence. Washington, DC: Department of Health and Human Services; 2002.
30. Garfinkel MS, Schumacher HR Jr, Husain A, et al. Evaluation of a yoga based regimen for treatment of osteoarthritis of the hands. J Rheumatol 1994;21(12):2341–3.
31. Haaz S, Bathon J, Bartlett S. Initial findings of an RCT of yoga on physical and psychological functioning in RA and OA [abstract]. Arthritis and Rheumatism Supplement 2007.
32. Haaz S, Bingham CO, Bathon JM, et al. The effect of yoga on clinical parameters in patients with rheumatoid arthritis [abstract]. Arthritis Rheum 2008;58(9):S893.
33. Haslock I, Monro R, Nagarathna R, et al. Measuring the effects of yoga in rheumatoid arthritis. Br J Rheumatol 1994;33(8):787–8.
34. Dash M, Telles S. Improvement in hand grip strength in normal volunteers and rheumatoid arthritis patients following yoga training. Indian J Physiol Pharmacol 2001;45(3):355–60.
35. Sharma M. Effects of a yoga intervention as a supportive therapy in arthritis. Yoga Studies 2005;412–6.
36. Badsha H, Chhabra V, Leibman C, et al. The benefits of yoga for rheumatoid arthritis: results of a preliminary, structured 8-week program. Rheumatol Int 2009;29(12):1417–21.
37. Bosch PR, Traustadottir T, Howard P, et al. Functional and physiological effects of yoga in women with rheumatoid arthritis: a pilot study. Altern Ther Health Med 2009;15(4):24–31.
38. Evans S, Moieni M, Taub R, et al. Iyengar yoga for young adults with rheumatoid arthritis: results from a mixed-methods pilot study. J Pain Symptom Manage 2010; 39(5):904–13.
39. Kolasinski SL, Garfinkel M, Tsai AG, et al. Iyengar yoga for treating symptoms of osteoarthritis of the knees: a pilot study. J Altern Complement Med 2005;11(4): 689–93.
40. Swanson RA, Holton EF. Research in organizations: foundations and methods of inquiry. San Francisco (CA): Bennett-Koehler Publishers; 2005.
41. Okolo EN. Health research design and methodology. Danvers (MA): CRC Press; 1991.
42. Osbourne JW, Costello AB. Sample size and subject to item ratio in principle component analysis. Practical Assessment, Research and Evaluation 2004;9(11).
43. Pedhazur EJ. Multiple regression in behavioral research: explanation and prediction. Fort Worth (TX): Harcourt Brace College Publishers; 1997.
44. Bosch PR, Traustadottirl T, Howard P, et al. Adaptation of the HPA axis to yoga in women with rheumatoid arthritis [abstract]. Arthritis Care Res (Hoboken) 2003.
45. Arambula P, Peper E, Kawakami M, et al. The physiological correlates of Kundalini Yoga meditation: a study of a yoga master. Appl Psychophysiol Biofeedback 2001;26(2):147–53.
46. Felson DT, Anderson JJ, Boers M, et al. The American College of Rheumatology preliminary core set of disease activity measures for rheumatoid arthritis clinical trials. The committee on outcome measures in rheumatoid arthritis clinical trials. Arthritis Rheum 1993;36(6):729–40.
47. Pham T, van der HD, Lassere M, et al. Outcome variables for osteoarthritis clinical trials: the OMERACT-OARSI set of responder criteria. J Rheumatol 2003;30(7): 1648–54.

48. Paulus HE, Ramos B, Wong WK, et al. Equivalence of the acute phase reactants C-reactive protein, plasma viscosity, and Westergren erythrocyte sedimentation rate when used to calculate American College of Rheumatology 20% improvement criteria or the Disease Activity Score in patients with early rheumatoid arthritis. Western Consortium of Practicing Rheumatologists. J Rheumatol 1999; 26(11):2324–31.

49. Salaffi F, Peroni M, Ferraccioli GF. Discriminating ability of composite indices for measuring disease activity in rheumatoid arthritis: a comparison of the Chronic Arthritis Systemic Index, Disease Activity Score and Thompson's articular index. Rheumatology (Oxford) 2000;39(1):90–6.

50. Haugen IK, Slatkowsky-Christensen B, Lessem J, et al. The responsiveness of joint counts, patient-reported measures and proposed composite scores in hand osteoarthritis: analyses from a placebo-controlled trial. Ann Rheum Dis 2010;69(8):1436–40.

51. Gilbert JC, Knowlton RG. Simple method to determine sincerity of effort during a maximal isometric test of grip strength. Am J Phys Med 1983;62(3):135–44.

52. Jones G, Cooley HM, Bellamy N. A cross-sectional study of the association between Heberden's nodes, radiographic osteoarthritis of the hands, grip strength, disability and pain. Osteoarthritis Cartilage 2001;9(7):606–11.

53. Giampaoli S, Ferrucci L, Cecchi F, et al. Hand-grip strength predicts incident disability in non-disabled older men. Age Ageing 1999;28(3):283–8.

54. Ware JE. Measuring patients' views: the optimum outcome measure. BMJ 1993; 306(6890):1429–30.

55. Meenan RF, Mason JH, Anderson JJ, et al. AIMS2. The content and properties of a revised and expanded Arthritis Impact Measurement Scales Health Status Questionnaire. Arthritis Rheum 1992;35(1):1–10.

The Role and Effect of Complementary and Alternative Medicine in Systemic Lupus Erythematosus

Anan J. Haija, MD*, Steffan W. Schulz, MD

KEYWORDS

- Systemic lupus erythematosus
- Complementary and alternative medicine • Effectiveness

Systemic lupus erythematosus (SLE) is a chronic and relapsing autoimmune disorder involving immune dysregulation and chronic widespread inflammation. Manifestations can include malar, discoid, and photosensitive skin rashes, arthralgias and arthritis, constitutional symptoms, potentially widespread internal organ disease, including dysfunction of renal, pulmonary, cardiac, neurologic, and/or gastrointestinal systems, as well as autoantibody production most typically identified by the presence of an antinuclear antibody (ANA). Criteria have been established by the American College of Rheumatology (ACR) to combine both clinical and serologic traits to aide in diagnosis.

The disease manifestations of SLE vary widely from patient to patient and, thus, treatment options cover a wide spectrum. Strategies range from conservative measures, such as acetaminophen and nonsteroidal antiinflammatory drugs (NSAIDs) for joint pain, to topical steroid creams and careful use of sunblock for dermatologic manifestations, to more directed immunologic therapies that vary in their immunosuppressive potential. Complementary and alternative medicine (CAM) is also an increasingly common supplement to standardized treatment and the prevalence and details of its application in SLE are crucial for the rheumatologist to understand.

A NEED FOR ALTERNATIVE THERAPIES IN SLE?

Overall treatment of SLE requires a comprehensive, multidisciplinary approach to the patient's individual and unique needs that typically extend beyond the treatment of the disease's immunologic dysfunction. Complaints of pain, fatigue, constitutional

Division of Rheumatology, Hospital of the University of Pennsylvania, Philadelphia, PA, USA
* Corresponding author.
E-mail address: Anan.Abuel-Haija@uphs.upenn.edu

Rheum Dis Clin N Am 37 (2011) 47–62
doi:10.1016/j.rdc.2010.11.005
0889-857X/11/$ – see front matter. Published by Elsevier Inc.

symptoms, and psychiatric disturbances are often difficult for patients to articulate and for the physician to diagnose and treat. In addition, their existence may fall outside the domain of the expertise of the rheumatologist who often supplements the primary care provider as a general overseer of the patient's global health.

Specific identifiable needs of the SLE patient are very diverse. Widespread pain can occur in joints and muscles in the absence of other disease activity and challenge conventional pain management strategies. Arthritis and arthralgia occur in between 53% and 88% of patients with SLE; additional complications of tendonitis, avascular necrosis, and myalgias also occur.[1] Overall physical function in SLE has been shown to be worse than in healthy controls.[2] Clinical investigations have shown a high prevalence of chronic pain syndromes, such as fibromyalgia, in some populations of patients with SLE.[3–5]

Beyond pain, there are many other sources of distress for patients with SLE. Fatigue is strongly associated.[6] A review of 34 articles by the Ad Hoc Committee on SLE identified fatigue as among the most prevalent and disabling complications of SLE. The committee found that fatigue was strongly linked with comorbidities, such as depression, anxiety, and poor quality of life.[7,8] Depression and anxiety are also common sequelae of SLE. A 2009 study by Bachen and colleagues[9] found that in 236 white women with SLE, 65% were diagnosed with at least 1 major mood disorder (depression, general anxiety, bipolar disorder); major depression occurred in 47%. Other findings included a 6-fold increased prevalence of bipolar disorder, an 11-fold increased risk of obsessive compulsive disorder (OCD) and a 2.5-fold increased risk of panic disorder. Equally concerning results showed that patients, especially those with anxiety, OCD, and dysthymia, frequently did not disclose symptoms to their physicians. Neuropsychiatric manifestations are common and often nondescript, adversely affecting quality of life.[10]

Evidence can be found to support and to refute a relationship between quality of life and disease activity in lupus. Some investigators argue that quality of life in patients with SLE is not associated directly with disease activity.[11,12] This has been attributed by some to study design issues. It can be difficult to match control groups to patient groups because of variability of population size, culture, and other factors. However, others have demonstrated that the overall effect of pain and mental health issues, in addition to physical dysfunction, organ disease, side effects of medications, and the emotional and psychological burden of having a chronic disease, can be considerable. An interesting study from the University of Chicago compared 90 patients with SLE to other patients groups with adult chronic diseases such as diabetes mellitus, congestive heart failure, myocardial infarction, and major depression. Patients with SLE had perceptions of vitality and physical functioning similar to patients with chronic heart failure but fared worse in categories including mental health and social functioning.[13] A similar loss of quality of life is experienced by the pediatric patient with SLE, as children struggle to retain some sense of control of their lives.[14] A patient's self-esteem, vitality, self-perception of illness, and its effect on their daily life can be profoundly negative in SLE.[2,15] Some studies have shown that the more active the disease, the worse this can be.[16,17] Poorer mental functioning and quality of life has been shown to be directly related to higher disease activity and SLE Disease Activity Index (SLEDAI) scores in several studies.[17,18] Lupus patients can develop a large degree of learned helplessness that can have a further effect on morbidity and quality of life.[19] Patients see SLE as an unpredictable and potentially uncontrollable disease that can impede their pursuit of personal goals and an overall normal life.[9,20] The presence of chronic pain, specifically fibromyalgia, is also associated with poorer quality of life.[12,21] Most agree that SLE is associated with an overall reduced quality of life compared with healthy controls and on the importance of including quality of life as a measure in creating treatment strategies for patients with SLE.[22]

Social factors may also play an important role in disease activity and quality of life in SLE. Higher levels of SLE activity have been linked to poor social support and resources available to the patients.[23] Challenges in access to care, education levels, and social class have been linked to SLE activity in some studies[24] but not in others.[23]

All of these factors combine to create a set of patient needs that westernized allopathic medicine often does not meet. A study by Danoff-Burg and Friedberg[25] analyzing surveys completed by 112 patients with SLE found that 100% of respondents had at least 1 unmet need in the setting on conventional SLE management with 91% having at least 1 unmet psychosocial need (78.6% feeling it was a significantly unmet need). A similar Australian study of 233 patients with SLE found 94% had an unmet need; the top 2 unmet needs were fatigue management (81%) and pain control (73%).[26]

THE DEMOGRAPHICS OF CAM USE

Understanding the who and the why behind the use of CAM in SLE is based on the fact that patients seek supportive treatments in addition to the traditional therapy overseen by the rheumatologist to fill their unmet needs. Patients with SLE and autoimmune disorders in general use CAM more often than the general population.[27] The TRINATION study (a multicenter international study of patients with SLE in Canada, Great Brittan, and the United States) reported that patients with SLE who use CAM have a slightly reduced satisfaction and perception of conventional medicine; patient self-perception of illness is higher although patients are not necessarily sicker when measured by objective markers.[27] In another study of patients with SLE, the overall disease activity of SLE was negatively associated with general satisfaction of the health care system.[2]

Other studies have correlated CAM use in patients with SLE with poorer physical function,[28] higher cumulative disease damage,[29] and higher self-perception of disease activity.[27] The TRINATION study did not conclude that objective measures of disease activity are associated with rates of CAM use.[27] A patient's cultural beliefs influences their expectations of conventional medicine and their use of CAM, but studies performed in communities where CAM use is more prevalent continue to demonstrate a correlation between disease activity and CAM use. A Singapore study of 192 patients with SLE found that 128 used some form of CAM with 57% of users citing continued disease activity and need for relief as opposed to 42% whose CAM use was driven by preference alone.[30] An additional study showed CAM use in patients with SLE in Singapore was influenced by the presence of pain and arthritis, the degree of satisfaction with conventional care, self-perception of health, and overall cost.[31]

The TRINATION study assessing CAM use in 707 patients from England, Canada, and the United States found 352 (49.8%) admitted use of at least 1 CAM therapy to the same extent in all 3 countries.[27] A letter to the editor described 70 of 107 Mexican patients surveyed having used CAM[32]; another reported 52.6% of Mexican patients with SLE used 2 CAM remedies or more,[28] and a third stated that 43.1% of 445 patients surveyed had tried a CAM therapy.[29]

Studies have varied in the demographic characteristics they have identified as having been associated with CAM use. A study investigating the use of CAM among Hispanics found that in 179 patients with SLE, 63% used CAM. These users were more likely to be women (75%) and of lower income and education levels.[33] On the other hand, the TRINATION study found no difference in CAM use between various income levels and instead suggested CAM users were more likely to be younger and on average have more years of education.[27]

SPECIFIC PRACTICES OF COMPLEMENTARY MEDICINE IN SLE

The definition of CAM supported by the ACR is broadly defined and includes those treatments, products, and practices that fall outside the mainstream of traditional western allopathic medicine. They may range from being safe and effective to being unsafe and ineffective.[34] In this review, attention is given to those therapies not commonly associated with traditional rheumatology office visits. A thorough review of the literature included topics such as acupuncture, massage therapy, mind-body relaxation and biofeedback techniques, exercise and stretching therapy, herbal and vitamin supplements, and psychosocial counseling among others. The paucity of controlled research trials in many of these areas is noticeable and data in many of these areas are lacking. A reporting and analysis of those interventions that have been identified as commonly used among patients with SLE and have been either the subject of individual studies or analyzed in review is included in this article.

Acupuncture

Acupuncture is an important component of CAM; it is used for several rheumatologic conditions including SLE. Its effectiveness in pain management has been best demonstrated in patients with chronic back pain where reduction in use of nonopioid analgesics was achieved in a randomized controlled cross-over trial of 10 years duration.[35] Additional evidence supports using acupuncture for pain relief in knee osteoarthritis[36–40] and for short-term benefit in the management of fibromyalgia pain, fatigue, and anxiety.[41,42] Studies are consistent in demonstrating a strong safety profile and minimal side effects, although serious side effects have been reported.[43] Others have suggested that reporting of adverse events has not been comprehensive enough, as shown by the Consolidated Standards of Reporting Trials (CONSORT).[44]

Clinical trials demonstrating positive results of acupuncture in fibromyalgia and osteoarthritis are encouraging because of the potential they suggest for treating pain, fatigue, and psychological disturbances commonly seen in patients with SLE. Unfortunately, there is very limited literature exploring the use of acupuncture in SLE directly. Greco and colleagues'[45] randomized controlled trial used 3 comparison groups: usual medical care alone, with acupuncture, or with minimal needling. The study chose outcome measures that included pain, fatigue, disease activity, and serologic levels of inflammatory cytokines. The trial suggested superiority of acupuncture and minimal needling over usual medical care alone. However, it did not demonstrate that sham acupuncture was inferior to true acupuncture. The study acknowledged the lack of statistical significance but suggested the true benefits were not seen in part because of inadequate sample size and power. Although side effects in Greco and colleagues' study were higher (23%, or 33 incidents, in 144 acupuncture sessions) than in previous studies, most adverse events were minor and ranged from pain during needle insertion and local bruising to dizziness and lightheadedness.

There were no serious adverse events in this trial, as has been the case in most published acupuncture studies. However, because acupuncture has not been shown to be efficacious specifically in SLE and is not widely covered by insurance plans, it is not often used. Further studies will be needed before rheumatologists can suggest acupuncture as a reasonable option for manifestations of lupus.

Meditation and Yoga

Mind-body techniques are commonly used CAM strategies that can provide the patient with a sense of some control of their disease. Included in this topic are the practices of meditation, yoga, and tai chi. Specific studies looking at the effect of meditation and tai chi on SLE activity are lacking, but there are studies detailing its use in other chronic medical illnesses. Reports on meditative prayer, Kundalini yoga, Sahaja yoga, Hatha yoga, mindfulness, and relaxation techniques are available.[46]

Yoga has been shown to be effective in controlling symptoms in several chronic conditions. In a large review from Arias and colleagues,[46] 82 studies were examined to analyze the efficacy and safety of meditative practices in treating medical illnesses. The review concluded that there is potential efficacy of meditative practices in treating nonpsychotic mood disturbances and anxiety disorders. Some evidence also suggests that relaxation techniques may be helpful for symptoms of menopausal and premenstrual syndrome. Yoga has been shown to have some positive effects with different strength of evidence in epilepsy, depression, OCD, opiate dependence, and sleep disturbance in patients with cancer. In a prospective randomized trial on epilepsy management, Panjwani and colleagues[47] reported changes in some of the electrophysiologic responses studied in patients with epilepsy who included auditory evoked potentials and visual contrast sensitivity. In a second epilepsy study, the same author randomized a group of 32 subjects to yoga for 6 months or to a control group. Those who practiced yoga had a reduction in electrocardiograph changes consistent with seizures.[48] Another study focused on yoga in patients with depression. Janakiramaiah and colleagues[49] reported a randomized study that compared yoga breath work to therapies for depression such as medications and electroconvulsive therapy (ECT). Woolery and colleagues[50] reported a short-term improvement in depression symptoms in mildly depressed young adults. One study on patients with OCD showed improvement in symptoms was more likely in patients practicing yoga than mindfulness meditation.[51]

To date, studies have not shown consistent reproducible results nor have they used randomized, placebo-, or sham-controlled designs. Many have lacked objective outcome measures. Nonetheless, side effects such as depersonalization have been very rarely reported,[52,53] Yoga has not been specifically evaluated in SLE. However, lupus shares unmet needs of disturbed psychosocial functioning and fatigue common with other chronic illnesses.[46] Until studies involving patients with SLE have been performed, yoga cannot be recommended for treatment of the manifestations of SLE.

Counseling, Behavioral Therapy, and Stress Management

An extension of mind-body interventions can include cognitive and behavioral therapies and several studies have investigated the benefit of psychosocial support provided to patients with SLE.[2,11,54] The previously mentioned study by Moses and colleagues[26] found that 6 of the top 10 unmet needs of patients with SLE were psychological, spiritual, or social in nature. Another study found 78.6% of 112 patients with SLE surveyed had unmet anxiety and social support needs; 70.5% felt there was an unmet need in depression management.[25] Poor disease coping, especially passive coping strategies, focusing on self-blame and wishful thinking, are present in SLE and associated with worse psychological and function status.[55] Those patients lacking psychosocial support and self-efficacy have higher self-reported disease activity.[56] Another study correlated lower socioeconomic status of patients with SLE with higher rates of depression and association with poorer mental and physical functioning.[57]

The last few years have seen more focused studies investigating the benefits of various counseling methods, including creating social networks for coping, 1-on-1 education sessions, stress reduction, and behavioral and psychological therapies for anxiety and depression. Patients with SLE receiving generalized social support and counseling show improved self-reporting of physical function, body pain, social function, and vitality.[2,18] Such counseling and education have a positive effect on overall disease management.[56] Counseling may have a buffering effect on disease activity, resulting in improved pain and fatigue.[58] An interesting study from Bae and colleagues[59] analyzed which demographic characteristics of patients with SLE would improve most with better social support resources. They found the greatest effect was in patients already above the poverty line; this study concluded that social support and counseling are most beneficial in those who already have financial and social advantages.

Counseling is included in this review as an alternative therapy because it serves to supplement cognitive and behavioral therapy in improving coping strategies in patients with SLE. Counseling involves either individual or group sessions and focuses most often on coping strategies and stress reduction. Studies of group counseling on disease and drug education, exercise, coping strategies, and stress reduction have found overall improvement in quality of life. These same studies, however, note no association between improvement and disease activity.[60,61] A study by Karlson and colleagues[62] reported that counseling sessions aimed at improving education, social support, and problem solving for patients with SLE and their spouses had a sustained effect on self-efficacy, mental health, and overall fatigue 12 months after the initial intervention. In a study of 8 patients by Maisiak and colleagues,[63] counseling was provided by telephone. Significant psychological benefit was found using the Arthritis Impact Measurement Scale in subjects receiving counseling by phone compared with those receiving standard care. Telephone-based counseling was used in another study of 58 patients with SLE and improvements in self-reported physical function and social support were seen.[64] In 1 unique study in which the phone interviewers themselves had SLE, providing counseling to other patients with SLE had a positive effect on overall well-being.[65] One may conclude from such studies that encouraging participation in local support groups may have an effect on a patient's cognitive health even if the effect on the disease process itself is negligible.

Several studies have focused more specifically on treating depression and anxiety in SLE. Groups focusing on education and coping strategies for anxiety and stress[66,67] and cognitive behavioral therapy[68] both demonstrated improvements in overall psychological function and self-esteem. An individual case report examining 1-on-1 psychotherapy in SLE showed improvement in self-identity and function.[69] Supportive-expressive group therapy was tested in a study from McGill University on 133 female patients with SLE with outcomes measuring quality of life, disease activity, and overall distress. The therapy was associated with some improvement in coping and overall distress, but a definitive benefit to the group could not be demonstrated.[70] The technique was used in a second study that focused on the potential effect on life domains, defined as relationship, intimacy, and instrumental life, such as work. Fifty-eight patients with SLE were assigned to therapy and compared with 66 patients with SLE in usual care. Significant and sustained improvements were noted in illness intrusiveness into the life domains of relationships and partner intimacy.[71]

Studies investigating the benefit of cognitive and behavioral therapies in SLE have been limited by small sample size and inadequate control groups. Results have been conflicting but these techniques have generally been shown to improve quality of life.

Exercise Therapy

Exercise is a useful tool in all patients to improve cardiovascular fitness, decrease metabolic abnormalities, reduce insulin resistance, reduce fatigue, and improve quality of life through pain reduction. Exercise is especially important for patients with SLE given their heightened susceptibility to cardiovascular events, as are modification of risk factors such as hyperlipidemia, hypertension, diabetes, sedentary lifestyle, and smoking. The mean age of the first myocardial infarction for patients with SLE is 49 years, significantly earlier than healthy controls.[72] Risks of low bone density are higher in patients with SLE[73] as are risks of fractures. Pain, fatigue, depression, and poor sleep in SLE can also result in poorer efforts toward physical activity.[74,75]

Patients with SLE have demonstrated worse exercise capacity and strength than sedentary healthy controls.[76] Tench and colleagues[75] compared a group of patients with SLE to matched normal controls and found that they have less aerobic fitness and reduced muscle strength unrelated to disease activity.

Several studies support use of exercise in SLE.[74,77] Low physical activity is associated with increased high-density lipoprotein and atherosclerosis in SLE. Increased strenuous exercise may reduce the risk of atherosclerosis in patients with SLE.[78] Cardiovascular exercise programs have also been shown to be effective in improving quality of life.[79] Bone loss can be attenuated in SLE with regular aerobic activity.[80] Inflammatory cytokines, including interleukin-6 and C-reactive protein, decrease in obese patients after exercise,[81] and these antiinflammatory effects of exercise that could be of interest in autoimmune disease. Exercise may also improve poor sleep[82] and is helpful in managing pain syndromes like fibromyalgia,[83] both often seen in SLE. Although there are no prospective randomized controlled trials, pilot studies suggest that exercise helps with fatigue in SLE.[84–86]

Vitamins and Dietary Supplements

Dihydroepiandrosterone

Low levels of dihydroepiandrosterone (DHEA) are seen in conditions such as aging, cardiovascular disease,[87,88] and SLE. Small studies have been done to determine the efficacy of DHEA supplementation in patients with SLE. In 1 open-label study,[89] DHEA was used in 10 patients with SLE for 3 to 6 months. Outcome measures included the SLEDAI score and physician's overall assessment. DHEA 200 mg daily was associated with improved SLEDAI scores and decreased glucocorticoid requirements. A subsequent double-blind randomized trial in 191 patients with SLE confirmed that DHEA supplementation could be associated with a modest stabilization of disease and reduction in steroid dose.[90] The most frequently noted side effect was mild acneiform dermatitis; no serious adverse events were associated with DHEA.

Another study done in 2005 by Nordmak and colleagues[91] analyzed the effect of DHEA in patients with SLE treated with glucocorticoids to evaluate efficacy on health-related quality of life. Patients were randomized to receive either DHEA or placebo for 6 months; subsequently, all patients were given DHEA. Health-related quality of life was assessed at baseline, 6, and 12 months using 4 validated questionnaires. The subjects' partners completed a questionnaire assessing mood and behavior at 6 months. Results demonstrated DHEA treatment increased serum levels of sulfated DHEA to normal levels. The DHEA group improved in SF-36 role emotional score and the HSCL-56 total score. The placebo group improved after subsequent DHEA treatment in the SF-36 mental health domain. Both groups improved in McCoy's Sex Scale during active treatment. There were no serious side effects reported.

A double-blinded, randomized, placebo-controlled clinical trial was conducted in 2009 to evaluate the effects of DHEA on fatigue and well-being in women with quiescent SLE by Hartkamp and colleagues.[92] Sixty women with quiescent lupus were randomized to receive oral DHEA 200 mg or placebo. Outcome parameters of general fatigue, depressed mood, mental well-being, and physical functioning were assessed before, during, and after treatment. Both groups improved nearly equally in the categories of general fatigue and mental well-being. The strong response of the placebo group suggested that the belief in taking DHEA was a stronger predictor for improvement than any differential effect of DHEA itself.

Studies to date have suggested a limited effect of DHEA on SLE activity and they are limited in sample size. Larger double-blind, placebo-controlled, randomized trials will be necessary to decide whether DHEA has a significant role in the treatment of lupus.

Fish oil

Fish oil has found use as a dietary supplement in conditions such as hypertriglyceridemia and IgA nephropathy. Data on SLE are limited.

One prospective, double-blind, cross-over study[93] assessed the effects of a diet low in fat and high in fish oil in 27 patients with active SLE treated for 34 weeks. Fourteen patients receiving marine oil improved in self-assessed daily function, whereas 13 patients receiving placebo (20 g olive oil) were rated as worse or no change. Another double-blind, double placebo-controlled trial was performed on 52 patients with SLE.[94] Two out of the 4 groups in the trial received 1 g fish oil daily and disease activity was measured by the revised Systemic Lupus Activity Measure (SLAM-R). The treatment group demonstrated significant improvement in SLAM-R scores. No effect was seen on hematologic, biochemical, and immunologic indices measured at baseline and 6, 12, and 24 weeks.

Another study[95] randomized patients to 2 double-blinded groups for 24 weeks: 1 received placebo, the other 3 g of fish oil daily. Disease activity was measured with the SLAM-R and British Isles Lupus Assessment Group (BILAG) index at baseline and the investigators found a statistically significant improvement 24 weeks in SLAM-R and BILAG. This was accounted for largely by improvement in constitutional, neuromotor, integument, and joint scores.

Vitamin D

Reports have suggested that patients with SLE have lower levels of vitamin D than healthy controls.[96,97] It is unknown why this seems to be the case. One study demonstrated a slightly higher incidence (although not statistically significant) of autoantibodies against vitamin D in a small SLE patient population.[98] A study of pediatric patients with SLE demonstrated lower vitamin D levels in general and an association with heightened disease activity in particular.[99]

Lower vitamin D levels in SLE were also seen in a study of the interaction of SLE disease activity and bone metabolism.[100] Comparisons were made between 2 groups of patients with SLE classified as high activity or minimal activity by SLEDAI scores. The group labeled as having high activity had statistically significantly lower vitamin D, osteocalcin, and bone-specific alkaline phosphatase levels. Although disease activity may contribute, sun avoidance, and the use of sunscreen may account for low vitamin D levels.[101] Predictors for low vitamin D in patients with SLE reported elsewhere include the presence of renal disease and photosensitivity.[97]

Although the importance of assessing vitamin D levels in SLE is crucial for maintenance of overall bone health, the effect of supplementing vitamin D on SLE activity is not known. Exploring the causes of deficiency and effects of replacement will require studies that include larger numbers of patients and tracking vitamin D levels before, during, and after disease flares.

Other vitamins

Vitamin C is a common dietary supplement. A popular use is reducing the severity of the common cold.

Several trials have investigated the use of vitamin C in SLE. In 1999, Minami and colleagues[102] showed that dietary nutrients may modify the clinical course of the disease in female patients with SLE, and that vitamin C intake is inversely associated with the risk of active disease. In the study, disease activity was evaluated based on the Lupus Activity Criteria Count. Patients were followed for 4 years and the study included 279 female patients. The study concluded that vitamin C may reduce SLE activity. The trial is limited in its poor estimation of the dosage requirements because the nutrient goal was estimated only by a semi-quantitative food frequency questionnaire. In addition, there is no indication of taking a specific vitamin C dose, and the conclusion was based on revealing an inverse association of intake of vitamin C with the risk of active disease.

Tam and colleagues[103] conducted a study in 2005 to evaluate the effects of long-term antioxidant vitamins on markers of oxidative stress and antioxidant defense and endothelial function in 39 patients with SLE. The patients were randomized into 2 groups, 1 receiving placebo and the other receiving vitamin C 500 mg and vitamin E 800 IU for 12 weeks. Markers were measured for oxidative stress and included malondialdehyde and allantoin. Antioxidants measured included erythrocyte superoxide dismutase, glutathione peroxidase, ascorbic acid, and vitamin E concentrations. Endothelial function was assessed by flow-mediated dilatation of the brachial artery and plasma concentration of von Willebrand factor and plasminogen activator inhibitor type 1. After treatment for 12 weeks, plasma ascorbic acid and α-tocopherol concentrations were significantly increased in the vitamin-treated group, and 1 oxidative stress marker, malondialdehyde, was significantly decreased. All other markers were unchanged. The study is limited in its effect because it was conducted for only 12 weeks and it did not look at clinical outcomes.

Weinmann and Hermann[104] conducted a study in a SLE mouse model (MRL/lpr) to study the potential of the antioxidant vitamin E to modulate the progress of SLE. Mice were supplemented with vitamin E 0.4 mg daily 5 times per week from 8 weeks of age onwards and compared with mice on a vitamin E–deficient diet. Supplementation with vitamin E extended the mean survival time from 157 to 196 days, and reduced the massive spleen and lymph node enlargement, titers of anti–double-stranded DNA antibodies and proteinuria. How this translates into humans is unclear. A double-blind, randomized, placebo-controlled trial is needed, keeping in mind that a judgment about affecting clinical outcomes needs good definition of these outcomes and adequate trial length to allow appropriate assessment of the frequencies of different organ involvement.

PRACTICALITY AND EFFECTIVENESS OF CAM IN THE PATIENT WITH SLE

Truly judging the full potential benefit of CAM and feeling comfortable recommending it is best done on an individual basis taking into consideration the unique presentation of SLE in the user along with their personal beliefs, education, finances, and so on. Overall, the TRINATION study concluded that CAM use in SLE did not significantly affect disease activity but also did not seem to cause poorer outcomes either.[27] The TRINATION study went on to suggest CAM did not reduce the use of conventional therapy but made it more likely patients would comply with conventional medicines. It seems physicians should not view CAM as a threat to take the place of traditional immunomodulatory therapies but as an adjunct that could be effective if used in the right clinical context in the correctly identified patient.

To find the appropriate role for CAM in SLE requires the rheumatologist to have knowledge of the various therapies and acceptance of the patient's desire to use them. The first hurdle is to ensure the patient is aware of the physician's interest in knowing about CAM use to avoid demonstrating a poor attitude toward the topic. In a Dutch study, 13% of CAM users were afraid they would receive negative feedback from their rheumatologist with regard to CAM.[105] Seventy-nine percent of an urban Hispanic population using CAM did not report the therapies to their doctor.[33] Physician ignorance is unlikely to reduce the usage of CAM and lack of an open dialog with patients will delay the rheumatologist from identifying problems with therapies they are not aware the patient is using. Identifying usage can also let the physician direct the patient toward more reputable therapies, as much variation does exist in the manufacturing and quality of products, the training of counselors, and overall safety of which patients may not be aware.

SUMMARY

The use of CAM is common among patients with SLE, especially those with active disease who often have poorer quality of life and significant unmet needs. It is important for the rheumatologist to be aware of these therapies and to ask the patient with SLE about their active use or future interest in CAM. Future studies on the effectiveness of the aforementioned therapies will be crucial to find better ways for the rheumatologist to integrate their use into the care of the patient with SLE.

REFERENCES

1. Wallace DJ. The musculoskeletal system. In: Hahn BH, editor. Dubois' lupus erythematosus. 6th edition. Philadelphia: Lippincott Williams & Wilkins; 2002. p. 629–44.
2. Sutcliffe N, Clarke AE, Levinton C, et al. Associates of health status in patients with systemic lupus erythematosus. J Rheumatol 1999;26(11):2352–6.
3. Buskila D, Press J, Abu-Shakra M. Fibromyalgia in systemic lupus erythematosus: prevalence and clinical implications. Clin Rev Allergy Immunol 2003;25(1):25–8.
4. Staud R. Are patients with systemic lupus erythematosus at increased risk for fibromyalgia? Curr Rheumatol Rep 2006;8(6):430–5.
5. Friedman AW, Tewi MB, Ahn C, et al. Systemic lupus erythematosus in three ethnic groups: XV. Prevalence and correlates of fibromyalgia. Lupus 2003;12(4):274–9.
6. Goligher EC, Pouchot J, Brant R, et al. Minimal clinically important difference for 7 measures of fatigue in patients with systemic lupus erythematosus. J Rheumatol 2008;35(4):635–42.
7. Ad Hoc Committee on Systemic Lupus Erythematosus Response Criteria for Fatigue. Measurement of fatigue in systemic lupus erythematosus: a systematic review. Arthritis Rheum 2007;57(8):1348–57.
8. Omdal R, Waterloo K, Koldingsnes W, et al. Fatigue in patients with systemic lupus erythematosus: the psychosocial aspects. J Rheumatol 2003;30(2):283–7.
9. Bachen EA, Chesney MA, Criswell LA. Prevalence of mood and anxiety disorders in women with systemic lupus erythematosus. Arthritis Rheum 2009;61(6):822–9.

10. Freire EA, Maia IO, Nepomuceno JC, et al. Damage index assessment and quality of life in systemic lupus erythematosus patients (with long-term disease) in Northeastern Brazil. Clin Rheumatol 2007;26(3):423–8.
11. McElhone K, Abbott J, Teh LS. A review of health related quality of life in systemic lupus erythematosus. Lupus 2006;15(10):633–43.
12. Kuriya B, Gladman DD, Ibañez D, et al. Quality of life over time in patients with systemic lupus erythematosus. Arthritis Rheum 2008;59(2):181–5.
13. Jolly M. How does quality of life of patients with systemic lupus erythematosus compare with that of other common chronic illnesses? J Rheumatol 2005;32(9): 1706–8.
14. Moorthy LN, Robbins L, Harrison MJ, et al. Quality of life in paediatric lupus. Lupus 2004;13(4):234–40.
15. Maeshima E, Maeshima S, Mizobata R, et al. Life-style activities in systemic lupus erythematosus. Clin Exp Rheumatol 2007;25(2):189–94.
16. Ward MM, Marx AS, Barry NN. Psychological distress and changes in the activity of systemic lupus erythematosus. Rheumatology 2002;41(2):184–8.
17. Mok CC, Ho LY, Cheung MY, et al. Effect of disease activity and damage on quality of life in patients with systemic lupus erythematosus: a 2-year prospective study. Scand J Rheumatol 2009;38(2):121–7.
18. Zheng Y, Ye DQ, Pan HF, et al. Influence of social support on health-related quality of life in patients with systemic lupus erythematosus. Clin Rheumatol 2009;28(3):265–9.
19. Engle EW, Callahan LF, Pincus T, et al. Learned helplessness in systemic lupus erythematosus: analysis using the rheumatology attitudes index. Arthritis Rheum 1990;33(2):281–6.
20. Dobkin PL, Da Costa D, Dritsa M, et al. Quality of life in systemic lupus erythematosus patients during more and less active disease states: differential contributors to mental and physical health. Arthritis Care Res 1999;12(6): 401–10.
21. Gladman DD, Urowitz MB, Gough J, et al. Fibromyalgia is a major contributor to quality of life in lupus. J Rheumatol 1997;24(11):2145–8.
22. Gladman D, Urowitz M, Fortin P, et al. Systemic lupus international collaborating clinics conference on assessment of lupus flare and quality of life measures in SLE. Systemic Lupus International Collaborating Clinics Group. J Rheumatol 1996;23(11):1953–5.
23. Ward MM, Lotstein DS, Bush TM, et al. Psychosocial correlates of morbidity in women with systemic lupus erythematosus. J Rheumatol 1999;26(10):2153–8.
24. Sutcliffe N, Clarke AE, Gordon C, et al. The association of socio-economic status, race, psychosocial factors and outcome in patients with systemic lupus erythematosus. Rheumatology 1999;38(11):1130–7.
25. Danoff-Burg S, Friedberg F. Unmet needs of patients with systemic lupus erythematosus. Behav Med 2009;35(1):5–13.
26. Moses N, Wiggers J, Nicholas C. Persistence of unmet need for care among people with systemic lupus erythematosus: a longitudinal study. Qual Life Res 2008;17(6):867–76.
27. Moore AD, Petri MA, Manzi S, et al. The use of alternative medical therapies in patients with systemic lupus erythematosus. Trination Study Group. Arthritis Rheum 2000;43(6):1410–8.
28. Alvarez-Nemegyei J, Bautista-Botello A. Complementary or alternative therapy use and health status in systemic lupus erythematosus. Lupus 2009;18(2): 159–63.

29. Alvarez-Nemegyei J, Bautista-Botello A, Dávila-Velázquez J. Association of complementary or alternative medicine use with quality of life, functional status or cumulated damage in chronic rheumatic diseases. Clin Rheumatol 2009; 28(5):547–51.
30. Leong KP, Pong LY, Chan SP. Why lupus patients use alternative medicine. Lupus 2003;12(9):659–64.
31. Lee GB, Charn TC, Chew ZH, et al. Complementary and alternative medicine use in patients with chronic diseases in primary care is associated with perceived quality of care and cultural beliefs. Fam Pract 2004;21(6):654–60.
32. Ramos-Remus C, Gamez-Nava JI, Gonzalez-Lopez L, et al. Use of alternative medicine in a consecutive sample of patients with systemic lupus erythematosus. J Rheumatol 1997;24(12):2490–1.
33. Mikhail N, Wali S, Ziment I, et al. Use of alternative medicine among Hispanics. J Altern Complement Med 2004;10(5):851–9.
34. Panush RS, for the Complementary and Alternative Therapies Subcommittee of the Communications and Marketing Committee. American College of Rheumatology position statement: "complementary" and "alternative" therapies for rheumatic diseases. Atlanta (GA): American College of Rheumatology; 1998.
35. Ghoname EA, Craig WF, White PF, et al. Percutaneous electrical nerve stimulation for low back pain: a randomized crossover study. JAMA 1999;281(9): 818–23.
36. Scharf H, Mansmann U, Streitberger K, et al. Acupuncture and knee osteoarthritis. Ann Intern Med 2006;145:12–20.
37. Gaw AC, Chang LW, Shaw LC. Efficacy of acupuncture on osteoarthritic pain. A controlled, double-blind study. N Engl J Med 1975;293(8):375–8.
38. Takeda W, Wessel J. Acupuncture for the treatment of pain of osteoarthritic knees. Arthritis Care Res 1994;7(3):118–22.
39. Berman BM, Lao L, Langenberg P, et al. Effectiveness of acupuncture as adjunctive therapy in osteoarthritis of the knee: a randomized, controlled trial. Ann Intern Med 2004;141(12):901–10.
40. Vas J, Méndez C, Perea-Milla E, et al. Acupuncture as a complementary therapy to the pharmacological treatment of osteoarthritis of the knee: randomised controlled trial. BMJ 2004;329(7476):1216.
41. Deluze C, Bosia L, Zirbs A, et al. Electroacupuncture in fibromyalgia: results of a controlled trial. BMJ 1992;305(6864):1249–52.
42. Martin DP, Sletten CD, Williams BA, et al. Improvement in fibromyalgia symptoms with acupuncture: results of a randomized controlled trial. Mayo Clin Proc 2006;81(6):749–57.
43. Witt C, Brinkhaus B, Jena S, et al. Acupuncture in patients with osteoarthritis of the knee: a randomized trial. Arthritis Rheum 2006;54(11):3485–93.
44. Capili B, Anastasi JK, Geiger JN. Adverse event reporting in acupuncture clinical trials focusing on pain. Clin J Pain 2010;26(1):43–8.
45. Greco CM, Kao AH, Maksimowicz-McKinnon K, et al. Acupuncture for systemic lupus erythematosus: a pilot RCT feasibility and safety study. Lupus 2008; 17(12):1108–16.
46. Arias AJ, Steinberg K, Banga A, et al. Systematic review of the efficacy of meditation techniques as treatments for medical illness. J Altern Complement Med 2006;12(8):817–32.
47. Panjwani U, Selvamurthy W, Singh SH, et al. Effect of Sahaja yoga meditation on auditory evoked potentials (AEP) and visual contrast sensitivity (VCS) in epileptics. Appl Psychophysiol Biofeedback 2000;25(1):1–12.

48. Panjwani U, Selvamurthy W, Singh SH, et al. Effect of Sahaja yoga practice on seizure control & EEG changes in patients of epilepsy. Indian J Med Res 1996; 103:165–72.
49. Janakiramaiah N, Gangadhar BN, Naga Venkatesha Murthy PJ, et al. Antidepressant efficacy of Sudarshan Kriya Yoga (SKY) in melancholia: a randomized comparison with electroconvulsive therapy (ECT) and imipramine. J Affect Disord 2000;57(1–3):255–9.
50. Woolery A, Myers H, Sternlieb B, et al. A yoga intervention for young adults with elevated symptoms of depression. Altern Ther Health Med 2004;10(2):60–3.
51. Shannahoff-Khalsa DS, Ray LE, Levine S, et al. Randomized controlled trial of yogic meditation techniques for patients with obsessive-compulsive disorder. CNS Spectr 1999;4(12):34–47.
52. Shapiro DH Jr. Adverse effects of meditation: a preliminary investigation of long-term meditators. Int J Psychosom 1992;39(1–4):62–7.
53. Kennedy RB Jr. Self-induced depersonalization syndrome. Am J Psychiatry 1976;133(11):1326–8.
54. Dobkin PL, Fortin PR, Joseph L, et al. Psychosocial contributors to mental and physical health in patients with systemic lupus erythematosus. Arthritis Care Res 1998;11(1):23–31.
55. McCracken LM, Semenchuk EM, Goetsch VL, et al. Cross-sectional and longitudinal analyses of coping responses and health status in persons with systemic lupus erythematosus. Behav Med 1995;20(4):179–87.
56. Karlson EW, Daltroy LH, Lew RA, et al. The relationship of socioeconomic status, race, and modifiable risk factors to outcomes in patients with systemic lupus erythematosus. Arthritis Rheum 1997;40(1):47–56.
57. Trupin L, Tonner MC, Yazdany J, et al. The role of neighborhood and individual socioeconomic status in outcomes of systemic lupus erythematosus. J Rheumatol 2008;35(9):1782–8.
58. Jump RL, Robinson ME, Armstrong AE, et al. Fatigue in systemic lupus erythematosus: contributions of disease activity, pain, depression, and perceived social support. J Rheumatol 2005;32(9):1699–705.
59. Bae SC, Hashimoto H, Karlson EW, et al. Variable effects of social support by race, economic status, and disease activity in systemic lupus erythematosus. J Rheumatol 2001;28(6):1245–51.
60. Sohng KY. Effects of a self-management course for patients with systemic lupus erythematosus. J Adv Nurs 2003;42(5):479–86.
61. Bricou O, Taïeb O, Baubet T, et al. Stress and coping strategies in systemic lupus erythematosus: a review. Neuroimmunomodulation 2006;13(5–6):283–93.
62. Karlson EW, Liang MH, Eaton H, et al. A randomized clinical trial of a psychoeducational intervention to improve outcomes in systemic lupus erythematosus. Arthritis Rheum 2004;50(6):1832–41.
63. Maisiak R, Austin JS, West SG, et al. The effect of person-centered counseling on the psychological status of persons with systemic lupus erythematosus or rheumatoid arthritis: a randomized, controlled trial. Arthritis Care Res 1996; 9(1):60–6.
64. Austin JS, Maisiak RS, Macrina DM, et al. Health outcome improvements in patients with systemic lupus erythematosus using two telephone counseling interventions. Arthritis Care Res 1996;9(5):391–9.
65. Peterson MG, Horton R, Engelhard E, et al. Effect of counselor training on skills development and psychosocial status of volunteers with systemic lupus erythematosus. Arthritis Care Res 1993;6(1):38–44.

66. Ng P, Chan W. Group psychosocial program for enhancing psychological well-being of people with systemic lupus erythematosus. J Soc Work Disabil Rehabil 2007;6(3):75–87.
67. Haupt M, Millen S, Jänner M, et al. Improvement of coping abilities in patients with systemic lupus erythematosus: a prospective study. Ann Rheum Dis 2005;64(11):1618–23.
68. Greco CM, Rudy TE, Manzi S. Effects of a stress-reduction program on psychological function, pain, and physical function of systemic lupus erythematosus patients: a randomized controlled trial. Arthritis Rheum 2004;51(4):625–34.
69. Geiger I, Langewitz W. Psychotherapy in a patient with lupus erythematodes, a disease with an uncertain course. Ther Umsch 2007;64(10):581–4.
70. Dobkin PL, Da Costa D, Joseph L, et al. Counterbalancing patient demands with evidence: results from a pan-Canadian randomized clinical trial of brief supportive-expressive group psychotherapy for women with systemic lupus erythematosus. Ann Behav Med 2002;24(2):88–99.
71. Edworthy SM, Dobkin PL, Clarke AE, et al. Group psychotherapy reduces illness intrusiveness in systemic lupus erythematosus. J Rheumatol 2003;30(5):1011–6.
72. Borba E, Bonfa E. Dyslipoproteinemias in systemic lupus erythematosus: influence of disease activity and anticardiolipin antibodies. Lupus 1997;6(6):533–9.
73. Bultink I, Lems W, Kostense P, et al. Prevalence of and risk factors for low bone mineral density and vertebral fractures in patients with systemic lupus erythematosus. Arthritis Rheum 2005;52(7):2044–50.
74. Keyser RE, Rus V, Cade WT, et al. Evidence for aerobic insufficiency in women with systemic lupus erythematosus. Arthritis Rheum 2003;49(1):16–22.
75. Tench C, Bentley D, Vleck V, et al. Aerobic fitness, fatigue, and physical disability in systemic lupus erythematosus. J Rheumatol 2002;29(3):474–81.
76. Houghton KM, Tucker LB, Potts JE, et al. Fitness, fatigue, disease activity, and quality of life in pediatric lupus. Arthritis Rheum 2008;59(4):537–45.
77. Ayán C, Martín V. Systemic lupus erythematosus and exercise. Lupus 2007;16(1):5–9.
78. Volkmann ER, Grossman JM, Sahakian LJ, et al. Low physical activity is associated with proinflammatory high-density lipoprotein and increased subclinical atherosclerosis in women with systemic lupus erythematosus. Arthritis Care Res 2010;62(2):258–65.
79. Carvalho MR, Sato EI, Tebexreni AS, et al. Effects of supervised cardiovascular training program on exercise tolerance, aerobic capacity, and quality of life in patients with systemic lupus erythematosus. Arthritis Rheum 2005;53(6):838–44.
80. Kipen Y, Briganti E, Strauss B, et al. Three year followup of bone mineral density change in premenopausal women with systemic lupus erythematosus. J Rheumatol 1999;26:310–7.
81. Esposito K, Pontillo A, Di Palo C, et al. Effect of weight loss and lifestyle changes on vascular inflammatory markers in obese women: a randomized trial. JAMA 2003;289(14):1799–804.
82. Da Costa D, Bernatsky S, Dritsa M, et al. Determinants of sleep quality in women with systemic lupus erythematosus. Arthritis Rheum 2005;53(2):272–6.
83. Häuser W, Klose P, Langhorst J, et al. Efficacy of different types of aerobic exercise in fibromyalgia syndrome: a systematic review and meta-analysis of randomised controlled trials. Arthritis Res Ther 2010;12(3):R79.
84. Robb-Nicholson LC, Daltroy L, Eaton H, et al. Effects of aerobic conditioning in lupus fatigue: a pilot study. Br J Rheumatol 1989;28(6):500–5.

85. Daltroy L, Robb-Nicholson C, Iversen M, et al. Effectiveness of minimally supervised home aerobic training in patients with systemic rheumatic disease. Br J Rheumatol 1995;34:1064–9.
86. Ramsey R, Schilling E, Dunlop D, et al. A pilot study on the effects of exercise in patients with systemic lupus erythematosus. Arthritis Care Res 2000;13(5): 262–9.
87. Derksen RH. Dehydroepiandrosterone (DHEA) and systemic lupus erythematosus. Arthritis Rheum 1998;27(6):335–47.
88. Lahita RG, Bradlow HL, Ginzler E, et al. Low plasma androgens in women with systemic lupus erythematosus. Arthritis Rheum 1987;30(3):241–8.
89. Van Vollenhoven RF, Engleman EG, McGuire JL. An open study of dehydroepiandrosterone in systemic lupus erythematosus. Arthritis Rheum 1994;37(9): 1305–10.
90. Petri MA, Lahita RG, Van Vollenhoven RF, et al. Effects of prasterone on corticosteroid requirements of women with systemic lupus erythematosus: a double-blind, randomized, placebo-controlled trial. Arthritis Rheum 2002; 46(7):1820–9.
91. Nordmark G, Bengtsson C, Larsson A, et al. Effects of dehydroepiandrosterone supplement on health-related quality of life in glucocorticoid treated female patients with systemic lupus erythematosus. Autoimmunity 2005; 38(7):531–40.
92. Hartkamp A, Geenen R, Godaert GL, et al. Effects of dehydroepiandrosterone on fatigue and well-being in women with quiescent systemic lupus erythematosus: a randomised controlled trial. Ann Rheum Dis 2010;69(6):1144–7.
93. Walton AJ, Snaith ML, Locniskar M, et al. Dietary fish oil and the severity of symptoms in patients with systemic lupus erythematosus. Ann Rheum Dis 1991;50(7):463–6.
94. Duffy EM, Meenagh GK, McMillan SA, et al. The clinical effect of dietary supplementation with omega-3 fish oils and/or copper in systemic lupus erythematosus. J Rheumatol 2004;31(8):1551–6.
95. Wright SA, O'Prey FM, McHenry MT, et al. A randomised interventional trial of omega-3-polyunsaturated fatty acids on endothelial function and disease activity in systemic lupus erythematosus. Ann Rheum Dis 2008;67(6):841–8.
96. Damanhouri LH. Vitamin D deficiency in Saudi patients with systemic lupus erythematosus. Saudi Med J 2009;30(10):1291–5.
97. Müller K, Kriegbaum NJ, Baslund B, et al. Vitamin D3 metabolism in patients with rheumatic diseases: low serum levels of 25-hydroxyvitamin D3 in patients with systemic lupus erythematosus. Clin Rheumatol 1995;14(4):397–400.
98. Bogaczewicz J, Sysa-Jedrzejowska A, Arkuszewska C, et al. [Prevalence of autoantibodies directed against 1,25(OH)2D3 in patients with systemic lupus erythematosus]. Pol Merkur Lekarski 2010;28(164):103–7 [in Polish].
99. Wright TB, Shults J, Leonard MB, et al. Hypovitaminosis D is associated with greater body mass index and disease activity in pediatric systemic lupus erythematosus. J Pediatr 2009;155(2):260–5.
100. Borba VZ, Vieira JG, Kasamatsu T, et al. Vitamin D deficiency in patients with active systemic lupus erythematosus. Osteoporos Int 2009;20(3):427–33.
101. Ruiz-Irastorza G, Egurbide MV, Olivares N, et al. Vitamin D deficiency in systemic lupus erythematosus: prevalence, predictors and clinical consequences. Rheumatology 2008;47(6):920–3.
102. Minami Y, Sasaki T, Arai Y, et al. Diet and systemic lupus erythematosus: a 4 year prospective study of Japanese patients. J Rheumatol 2003;30(4):747–54.

103. Tam LS, Li EK, Leung VY, et al. Effects of vitamins C and E on oxidative stress markers and endothelial function in patients with systemic lupus erythematosus: a double blind, placebo controlled pilot study. J Rheumatol 2005;32(2):275–82.
104. Weimann BJ, Hermann D. Inhibition of autoimmune deterioration in MRL/lpr mice by vitamin E. Int J Vitam Nutr Res 1999;69(4):255–61.
105. Visser GJ, Peters L, Rasker JJ. Rheumatologists and their patients who seek alternative care: an agreement to disagree. Br J Rheumatol 1992;31(7):485–90.

Mindfulness Meditation: A Primer for Rheumatologists

Laura A. Young, MD, PhD

KEYWORDS
- Fibromyalgia • Rheumatoid arthritis • Osteoarthritis
- Mindfulness meditation
- Mindfulness-based stress reduction (MBSR) • Stress

Meditation, with its origins rooted in ancient religious and spiritual practices dating back over centuries ago, has only in the past several decades begun to capture the attention of mainstream Western researchers and health care providers who are gradually beginning to value this mind-body practice as a tool to foster improved physiologic and psychological health.[1] In the current medical environment, it is not uncommon for patients to report the use of mind-body therapies as an adjunct to Western medical treatment.[2] Over the past decade, there has been an increasing interest in meditation as a mind-body approach, and in particular mindfulness meditation, given its potential to alleviate emotional distress and promote improved well being in a variety of populations.[3–5] The overall purpose of this review is to provide the practicing rheumatologist with an overview of mindfulness and how it can be applied to Western medical treatment plans to enhance both the medical and psychological care of patients.

WHAT IS MINDFULNESS?

The word mindfulness is derived from the Pali word *sati*, meaning "to remember," with secondary meanings of "attention" and "awareness." Remembering refers to reconnecting to the immediate moment of experience, not the recollection of a past event. A contemporary definition of mindfulness offered by Kabat-Zinn,[6] states that mindfulness is the awareness that emerges through, "paying attention on purpose, in the present moment, and non-judgmentally, to the unfolding of experience moment to moment." Similar descriptions are offered by other leaders in the field, including

This work was supported by Grant Number 5K23AT004946–02 from the National Institutes of Health.

Division of Endocrinology, Department of Internal Medicine, University of North Carolina School of Medicine, 8023 Burnett Womack Building, Campus Box # 7170 UNC-CH, Chapel Hill, NC 27599-7170, USA

E-mail address: Laura_Young@med.unc.edu

Rheum Dis Clin N Am 37 (2011) 63–75
doi:10.1016/j.rdc.2010.11.010
0889-857X/11/$ – see front matter © 2011 Elsevier Inc. All rights reserved.

"mindfulness is the nonjudgmental observation of the ongoing stream of internal and external stimuli as they arise" and "a receptive attention to and awareness of present events and experience."[7,8] Notably, two concepts pervade these descriptions of mindfulness: (1) holding one's attention in the present moment and (2) maintaining an attitude of acceptance, openness, and nonjudgment.[9] The validity of this two-component model has been debated; however, it still remains a useful, widely accepted definition.[10,11]

Mindfulness meditation (process) is a mental technique that is used to strengthen the capacity to establish and sustain mindful awareness (outcome).[12] The practice of mindful meditation cultivates attentional focus and stability by directing the mind to remain connected to the present moment experience. Attention is usually sustained by concentrating on the breath.[6] Participants are instructed to follow the flowing cycle of breathing with their full attention. Depending on the exercise, the focus of attention can vary and may include sensations in the body during rest or movement, a sound, or a visual focus, such as a candle flame or an image. Although the object of focus varies, in all instances, the goal of the practice is to train attention to remain fully engaged with the experience and remain in the present moment. Although this may seem simple, after attempting to keep attention focused for only a few moments, it is natural for novices to relate difficulty in maintaining focus on the present moment. Without training, attention drifts and becomes lost in memories of the past and thoughts of the future. With practice over time, remaining in the present becomes easier and is more likely to occur spontaneously. Meditation is simply a tool to assist in the acquisition of an awareness, which is broad, balanced, present focused, and behaviorally neutral.

HEALTH BENEFITS LINKED TO MINDFULNESS PRACTICE

A relatively wide collection of studies, of varying quality, in healthy people have linked mindfulness training to improvements in stress, anxiety, and depressed mood.[13–16] Mindfulness is also effective at decreasing stress and promoting positive mood states in patients with a variety of chronic health conditions.[17–28] Studies examining the effects of mindfulness training on traditional Western medicine outcomes, including morbidity and mortality, are beginning to emerge.[28] Data from the field of psychiatry and mental health show that mindfulness interventions can be efficacious in the treatment of mood disorders.[5,7,29] Furthermore, accumulating data support the notion that mindfulness meditation may ameliorate physiologic changes that accompany chronic mental and emotional stress, including improved cortisol secretion profiles and beneficial anatomic changes in the brain.[30,31] Although these early findings are encouraging, additional work examining psychological and physiologic changes that occur during and after mindfulness meditation training are clearly necessary.

PROPOSED MECHANISMS OF ACTION

Given the significant salutary effects of mindfulness training, the question remains, "what mechanisms are mediating these outcomes?"[5,7,31] The mechanisms through which mindfulness decreases stress and increases well being are not well understood; however, a variety of proposed mechanisms of action abound in the literature. Several of the more prominent theories will be briefly reviewed. One popular hypothesis is that the cultivation of mindfulness facilitates a fundamental shift in perspective, termed reperceiving.[11] Similar to decentering, reperceiving refers to observing one's thoughts and feelings as temporary emotion-neutral events occurring in the mind, which do not require judgment. Shapiro theorized that reperceiving leads to greater clarity, objectivity, and equanimity and facilitates improved self-regulation, values clarification, and cognitive and emotional flexibility.[11] However, empiric testing of this theory suggests that reperceiving and mindfulness are in fact overlapping constructs, and there is little support that reperceiving alone mediates improvements in psychological outcome variables.[32] Others speculate that it is the development of mindful awareness that mediates improved psychological outcomes.[33] In a group of novices, there was a positive relationship between the time spent practicing meditation and (1) the tendency to be mindful in daily life and (2) psychological improvements. Increased mindfulness in turn mediated the relationship between the time spent meditating and reductions in stress and improvements in psychological functioning.[34] Additional work supporting this concept showed that long-term meditation practice is associated with being able to describe one's internal experiences with words and being nonjudgemental and nonreactive toward them.[35] Furthermore, these key constructs of mindfulness were found to mediate the relationship between meditation experience (measured in months) and well being in experienced meditators. These findings support the notion that mindfulness is cultivated through meditation and may mediate the relationship between meditation practice and improved mental health.

Experimentally, changes in the ability to direct and manage attention have been demonstrated only after 5 days of mindfulness meditation training as well as after longer periods of training.[36,37] There are several proposed therapeutic benefits of maintaining a present-focused attention that is nonjudgemental and nonreactive. Self-focused attention, in the form of rumination, is linked to a variety of psychological maladies and poor outcomes. Rumination is the mental propensity to repetitively think about situations, thoughts, feelings, or emotions, which are typically of a negative nature. It has been theorized that the self-focused nature of the rumination is not harmful, rather it is how one processes these thoughts that predicts maladaptive outcomes. Sustaining a mindful self-focus that encourages a nonjudgmental nonreactive awareness of the present moment, even in people prone to rumination, promotes a mode of self-thought processing that is more adaptive.[38,39] Additional benefits of self-focused attention have been theorized, including increased mental flexibility, improved self-regulation, decreased emotional reactivity, and reduced avoidance.[24,40–42] For a more in-depth consideration of these issues, readers are directed to Baer's thoughtful review.[43]

COMMON METHODS USED TO TEACH MINDFULNESS

In this section, the authors briefly reviews the most common mindfulness approaches used by patients. The intent is to enable the practicing rheumatologist to make more informed recommendations to patients interested in incorporating mindfulness into their treatment plans. The completely secular nature of these approaches accommodates a wide audience. These interventions follow in the footsteps of earlier psychological approaches, including behavioral therapy and cognitive behavioral therapy (CBT). In stark contrast to CBT, in which the emphasis is on the use of cognitive restructuring of beliefs that mediate negative effect, the so-called third wave therapies promote the creation of a constructive relationship with disturbing emotions, which ultimately promotes acceptance.[44]

Mindfulness-Based Stress Reduction

Likely the most well-known and popular program designed to train participants in mindfulness, the Mindfulness-Based Stress Reduction (MBSR) program was developed in the 1970s by Jon Kabat-Zinn[24] at the University of Massachusetts. Initially developed as a behavioral intervention for patients with chronic pain and stress-related conditions, the MBSR program has expanded globally and can now be found in a variety of health care and community settings, including more than 400 hospital and medical schools in the United States.[21] MBSR is a standardized program conducted as an 8-week class with weekly sessions typically lasting for 2.5 to 3 hours. During the training, participants practice (1) sitting meditation using the breath as an anchor, (2) contemplative walking, (3) mindful movement through the use of gentle hatha-type yoga postures, and (4) the body scan in which attention control is practiced by systematically focusing on the sensations in various parts of the body. Near the end of the 8-week training program, application of mindful awareness to daily activities, often referred to as informal mindfulness practice, is encouraged. Mindfulness activities are practiced both in class and as homework. Audio recordings are provided to support home practice. Participants are expected to complete approximately 45 minutes of formal mindfulness practice at least 6 days per week during the 8-week period. During an all-day retreat near the end of the training, participants remain in silence and have the opportunity to practice their newly acquired mindfulness skills during a sustained and uninterrupted period of time. An essential component of the weekly classes includes discussion about the experiences that occur during the practice of mindfulness both in and out of the classroom. The effect of teacher experience, frequency of weekly session attendance, duration of home practice, and frequency of home practice likely affects the degree of symptomatic improvement reported by participants, but results have been mixed.[18,19,45–49] Patients can be referred to the Center for Mindfulness in Medicine, Healthcare, and Society at the University of Massachusetts for a listing of teachers who have completed standardized MBSR training (http://www.umassmed.edu/cfm/stress/index.aspx).

Mindfulness-Based Cognitive Therapy

Largely based on the concepts of mindfulness derived from MBSR, the focus of mindfulness-based cognitive therapy (MBCT) is on the treatment of depression rather than stress.[50] Specifically designed for use in the prevention of depression relapse, the theoretical foundation of MBCT rests on research showing that the individuals most vulnerable to depression relapse are those who have mood-related reactivation of negative thinking patterns and inappropriate responses to negative thoughts and emotions.[51–53] A combination of mindfulness training and cognitive therapy are used to cultivate a decentered approach to internal experience. Unlike traditional CBT exercises that attempt to change thoughts, in MBCT, the focus is on acceptance rather than change. Because this is a relatively new intervention, at present, there is no network of qualified providers. Creators of the intervention recommend using their book *The Mindful Way Through Depression* and/or working with a teacher or therapist who incorporates MBSR or other mindfulness practices into their work for those interested in this approach.[54]

Dialectical Behavior Therapy

Originally developed through insight gained while working with patients who had suicidal ideation and borderline personality disorder, dialectical behavior therapy (DBT) is a modified CBT program, drawing from principals in behavioral science, dialectical philosophy, and Zen meditation practice.[55] Therapists and clients work to balance change with acceptance. Traditional CBT helps the participant change inappropriate behaviors, thoughts, and emotions, whereas mindfulness training helps to facilitate acceptance and change. Participants are asked to make a 1-year commitment to the therapy. There are several components to DBT, including individual psychotherapy, group skills training, and telephone consultations between sessions. Readers are referred to the DBT training manual for a more in-depth review.[40]

CLINICAL APPLICATIONS OF MINDFULNESS SPECIFIC TO THE PRACTICING RHEUMATOLOGIST

Although there is a growing body of evidence supporting the use of mindfulness training as an adjunct to conventional therapy for a variety of medical and psychological conditions, studies specifically examining this intervention in patients with rheumatologic conditions are limited. The following discussion highlights several clinical concerns that are frequently encountered by the practicing rheumatologist for which mindfulness training may be beneficial.

Chronic Pain

Collectively, rheumatologic diseases have been classified to be the most prominent cause of chronic pain in the developed world.[56,57] Chronic pain is often associated with a multitude of challenges not only for the patient but also for the cadre of family, friends, and health care providers caring for them. Uncontrolled chronic pain can lead to poorer quality of life, disability, and psychosocial problems in patients with rheumatologic conditions.[58] Although most health care providers are aware of the role the mind-body connection has in partially mediating chronic pain symptoms, many feel underprepared and/or unqualified to make recommendations for therapeutic interventions intended to target this important symptom-modifying axis.[59,60] Although a wide range of mind-body therapies have been shown to be effective for the treatment of chronic pain and the inclusion of these interventions into comprehensive treatment plans has been recommended by consensus panels, only 20% of patients with chronic pain report the use of such adjunctive therapies.[61,62]

CBT is a widely used and accepted mind-body approach, which uses cognitive restructuring to modify maladaptive thoughts and behaviors related to pain; however, the overall reported effect sizes for CBT are generally small in patients with chronic pain.[63,64] Eliminating maladaptive thoughts may not be a realistic strategy in patients with rheumatologic conditions who suffer from chronic pain because most face continual daily reminders of their chronic medical problems. A more realistic approach may be the promotion of acceptance. Mindfulness-based approaches to pain management encourage participants to alter their relationships and reflexive behavioral responses to these maladaptive thoughts through nonjudgmental acceptance. Pain acceptance has been described as "a willingness to experience continuing pain without needing to reduce, avoid, or otherwise change it."[65] Experienced mindfulness practitioners demonstrate reduced anticipation and negative appraisal of pain under experimental conditions.[66] Higher degrees of mindfulness in patients with chronic pain are related to lower self-reported pain, emotional distress, disability, and use of pain medication.[67] Lower degrees of mindfulness are related to greater distorted thinking about pain, specifically pain catastrophizing, characterized by rumination about pain, feelings of hopelessness, and exaggeration of pain-related symptoms.[68]

Training in mindfulness, particularly through the use of MBSR, has been shown to be effective for the treatment of chronic pain originating from a variety of causes, although not all studies have shown positive results related to pain reduction.[21–26] A recent uncontrolled observational study suggests that participants enrolled in a community-based MBSR training program who reported chronic pain exhibited improvements in pain scores after completion of the course.[49] Participants with chronic neck/back pain and arthritis were most likely to have significant improvements in pain after the MBSR training, whereas those with fibromyalgia and chronic headache did not have significant improvement in self-reported pain, suggesting a potential role in certain patients with rheumatologic disease.

Some of the highest quality evaluations of mindfulness interventions in chronic pain have been in patients with rheumatoid arthritis (RA), osteoarthritis, and fibromyalgia. After 8 weeks of training, self-reported pain significantly improved in 144 participants with RA regardless of intervention (CBT vs mindfulness training vs disease education), although greater effects were seen with CBT and education compared with mindfulness training.[69] Mindfulness training did not positively affect patients' perceived control over their pain, whereas CBT and education showed beneficial effects. The relative value of the treatments in patients with RA varied based on depression history. Those with a history of two or more episodes of depression who completed mindfulness training were more likely to show improvements in pain-coping self-efficacy, pain catastrophizing, and physician-assessed joint tenderness and joint swelling. The data supporting the use of mindfulness in patients with pain due to osteoarthritis are less compelling. In two different heterogeneous groups of older adults with chronic low-back pain, in which a large proportion of the participants attributed the cause of their pain to osteoarthritis, the report of pain by those who had undergone MBSR training was not significantly different from those in the wait-list control or educational control conditions.[70,71] Chronic pain self-efficacy and disability scores improved in both the mindfulness and educational control groups.[71] In a randomized controlled trial of a mindfulness-based intervention for women with fibromyalgia, significant improvements in pain were noted for those in the mindfulness group compared with the wait-list control condition.[72] Similar findings were noted in 58 women with fibromyalgia participating in a quasi-randomized trial. Self-reported pain scores, pain perception, and the ability to cope with pain improved after an 8-week MBSR training compared with the support control group immediately after the intervention. Improvements were maintained over a 3-year follow-up time period.[73] In contrast, Astin and colleagues[74] showed similar improvements in pain in patients with fibromyalgia completing a mindfulness-based movement class compared with those in an educational control group. Although no conclusive recommendations can be made regarding the use of mindfulness interventions as an adjunctive means to control pain in patients with rheumatologic conditions, these initial findings suggest that mindfulness training does not cause harm.

Mental Health

The benefits of mindfulness training, particularly on depression and anxiety, have been repeatedly shown in a variety of populations, including in those with chronic medical conditions.[5,29,75–77] A more mindful awareness might buffer against the harmful influence of perceived stress on psychological well being, particularly in people who are susceptible to poor psychological functioning. Similar to other populations, improvements in mood have been shown to occur after mindfulness training in patients with rheumatologic conditions. In patients with RA, immediately after MBSR training, there were no notable improvements in psychological distress or depressive affect; however, 4 months after the intervention, improvements in psychological distress, but not depression, were noted.[46] In a second study of patients with rheumatoid arthritis, positive affect improved for both those receiving CBT and mindfulness, but the greatest improvements in both negative and positive affect were seen in those with a history of two or more episodes of depression, suggesting that those with recurrent depression were most responsive to the mindfulness intervention.[69] Modest improvements in psychological distress have been shown after completion of mindfulness training in patients with fibromyalgia compared with controls.[72] In a group of 91 women with fibromyalgia, Sephton and colleagues[78] showed specific improvements in depression in those who had mindfulness training compared to controls. Furthermore, mindfulness training in women with fibromyalgia has been shown to improve patients' sense of optimism and control over their life, which was related to lower depressive symptoms.[79] Mindfulness combined with a movement intervention was shown to be as efficacious as education and support in improving symptoms of depression in patients with fibromyalgia.[74] Observational data evaluating changes in depression and anxiety before and after MBSR training suggest that patients with fibromyalgia had small nonsignificant changes in psychological distress, whereas patients with arthritis had the largest improvements in psychological distress when compared with patients with other types of chronic pain.[49] Based on the data, a significant amount of work still needs to be done to evaluate the effect of mindfulness training on mental health in patients with rheumatologic conditions. MBCT, with its proven track record for depression relapse prevention, is a particularly appealing mindfulness approach for patients with rheumatologic disease given the high rates of clinically significant depression in these patients. MBCT has yet to be formally evaluated in a cohort with a specific rheumatologic disease. One word of caution to health care providers who may want to suggest mindfulness training as an adjunctive approach to a multidisciplinary care plan. Mindfulness interventions may not be appropriate for people who are actively suffering from acute clinical depression. It has been theorized that the intensity of negative thoughts, poor concentration, and restlessness, which often accompany an episode of acute depression, might make meaningful participation in mindfulness exercises difficult and uncomfortable. Developing the necessary attentional control skills may be challenging during a major depressive episode, although this long-held belief has recently been questioned.[80,81]

Immune Function

Accumulating data suggest that training in mindfulness meditation may also support improved physiologic functioning. Although the exact mechanisms remain largely unknown, it is hypothesized that mindfulness meditation may exert its favorable effects through a variety of pathways, including decreased sympathetic activation and improved neuroendocrine function, two pathways intimately coupled to immune function.[82] In a landmark study, Davidson and colleagues[47] demonstrated that training in mindfulness meditation enhanced antibody production after influenza vaccination in healthy adults. Extending this work to conditions in which immune dysfunction plays an important role, including cancer and human immunodeficiency virus (HIV) infection, has also yielded promising results. In patients with breast and prostate cancer, a shift from a proinflammatory response, to a more antiinflammatory response, after MBSR participation has been observed.[17,18] This shift from a proinflammatory state was maintained at the 1-year follow-up in this cohort of patients with breast and prostate cancer as evidenced by a continued decrease in Th1 cytokine production.[83] In HIV-positive individuals, notable increases in natural killer cell activity from baseline were noted after MBSR training.[84] In women with early-stage breast cancer not undergoing chemotherapy, those who underwent MBSR training displayed a restoration of natural killer cell activity and improvement in cytokine profiles, whereas those in the control group continued to show immune function abnormalities.[85] The investigators speculate that this favorable shift in immune function may be related to lower cortisol secretion in the MBSR group compared with the non-MBSR group. The relationship between improved psychological well being and improved immune function is less clear, with some studies showing a positive relationship between the two and others showing no association.[17,84,86] Although these findings are interesting, they are also preliminary and require confirmation in larger populations. To date, little work has been done on the impact of mindfulness training on immune function in patients with rheumatologic conditions. Two studies have evaluated the impact of mindfulness training on immune function in patients with RA and have shown no improvement in the Disease Activity Score (DAS), which includes a measure of the erythrocyte sedimentation rate, or IL-6 concentrations.[46,69] While the apparent beneficial effects of mindfulness training on certain immune function parameters are interesting, they are also preliminary, and require confirmation in larger populations.

SUMMARY

Although historically mindfulness meditation is ancient, as described in this review, research in the field is in its early stages but rapidly expanding in both quality and quantity. This expansion has been fueled in part by a 2007 Agency for Healthcare Research and Quality review that called into question the efficacy of meditation for improving health, which cited the rigor of the current studies of meditation as generally poor.[87] Nonetheless, it is clear that for many, mindfulness training can have powerful psychological and possibly physiologic effects. Many questions remain unanswered and further investigation is warranted. Studies of mindfulness demonstrate that training leads to improved quality of life in a wide variety of patient populations, including in patients with rheumatologic disease. Considering that decreased quality of life is common among people with chronic disease and given the generally benign nature of this behavioral intervention, it is perhaps surprising that mindfulness training is not recommended more often by health care providers in all fields. The clinical importance of improved quality of life as a predictor of morbidity and mortality is debated; however, it is difficult to not argue that part of our role as clinicians should be to encourage our patients to engage in activities that promote optimal enjoyment of life despite chronic medical conditions. We are quickly learning through the power of biomedical research what other cultures have recognized for thousands of years-mindfulness meditation is a powerful tool that can foster improved coping and growth. There is a great deal more that we need to learn, but it seems certain that mindfulness-based interventions have a future in both Western medicine and society.

REFERENCES

1. Ludwig DS, Kabat-Zinn J. Mindfulness in medicine. JAMA 2008;300(11):1350–2.
2. Barnes PM, Bloom B, Nahin RL. Complementary and alternative medicine use among adults and children: United States, 2007. Natl Health Stat Report 2008; 12:1–23.
3. Reibel DK, Greeson JM, Brainard GC, et al. Mindfulness-based stress reduction and health-related quality of life in a heterogeneous patient population. Gen Hosp Psychiatry 2001;23(4):183–92.
4. Chiesa A, Serretti A. Mindfulness-based stress reduction for stress management in healthy people: a review and meta-analysis. J Altern Complement Med 2009; 15(5):593–600.
5. Grossman P, Niemann L, Schmidt S, et al. Mindfulness-based stress reduction and health benefits. A meta-analysis. J Psychosom Res 2004;57(1):35–43.

6. Kabat-Zinn J. Full catastrophe living: using the wisdom of your body and mind to face stress, pain, and illness (15th Anniversary Ed.). New York: Delta Trade Paperback/Bantam Dell; 2005.
7. Baer RA. Mindfulness training as a clinical intervention: a conceptual and empirical review. Clinical psychology. Science and Practice 2003;10(2):125–43.
8. Brown KW, Ryan RM. The benefits of being present: mindfulness and its role in psychological well-being. J Pers Soc Psychol 2003;84(4):822–48.
9. Bishop SR, Lau M, Shapiro S, et al. Mindfulness: a proposed operational definition. Clinical psychology. Science and Practice 2004;11(3):230–41.
10. Hayes SC, Strosahl KD, Wilson KG. Acceptance and commitment therapy: an experiential approach to behavior change. New York: Guilford Press; 1999.
11. Shapiro SL, Carlson LE, Astin JA, et al. Mechanisms of mindfulness. J Clin Psychol 2006;62(3):373–86.
12. Shapiro SL, Carlson LE. The art and science of mindfulness: integrating mindfulness into psychology and the helping professions. Washington, DC: American Psychological Association; 2009.
13. Astin JA. Stress reduction through mindfulness meditation: effects on psychological symptomatology, sense of control, and spiritual experiences. Psychother Psychosom 1997;66(2):97–106.
14. Jain S, Shapiro SL, Swanick S, et al. A randomized controlled trial of mindfulness meditation versus relaxation training: effects on distress, positive states of mind, rumination, and distraction. Ann Behav Med 2007;33(1):11–21.
15. Klatt MD, Buckworth J, Malarkey WB. Effects of low-dose mindfulness-based stress reduction (MBSR-ld) on working adults. Health Educ Behav 2009;36(3):601–14.
16. Shapiro SL, Schwartz GE, Bonner G. Effects of mindfulness-based stress reduction on medical and premedical students. J Behav Med 1998;21(6):581–99.
17. Carlson LE, Speca M, Patel KD, et al. Mindfulness-based stress reduction in relation to quality of life, mood, symptoms of stress, and immune parameters in breast and prostate cancer outpatients. Psychosom Med 2003;65(4):571–81.
18. Carlson LE, Speca M, Patel KD, et al. Mindfulness-based stress reduction in relation to quality of life, mood, symptoms of stress and levels of cortisol, dehydroepiandrosterone sulfate (DHEAS) and melatonin in breast and prostate cancer outpatients. Psychoneuroendocrinology 2004;29(4):448–74.
19. Shapiro SL, Bootzin RR, Figueredo AJ, et al. The efficacy of mindfulness-based stress reduction in the treatment of sleep disturbance in women with breast cancer: an exploratory study. J Psychosom Res 2003;54(1):85–91.
20. Ledesma D, Kumano H. Mindfulness-based stress reduction and cancer: a meta-analysis. Psychooncology 2009;18(6):571–9.
21. Kabat-Zinn J, Lipworth L, Burney R. The clinical use of mindfulness meditation for the self-regulation of chronic pain. J Behav Med 1985;8(2):163–90.
22. Plews-Ogan M, Owens JE, Goodman M, et al. A pilot study evaluating mindfulness-based stress reduction and massage for the management of chronic pain. J Gen Intern Med 2005;20(12):1136–8.
23. Teixeira ME. Meditation as an intervention for chronic pain: an integrative review. Holist Nurs Pract 2008;22(4):225–34.
24. Kabat-Zinn J. An outpatient program in behavioral medicine for chronic pain patients based on the practice of mindfulness meditation: theoretical considerations and preliminary results. Gen Hosp Psychiatry 1982;4(1):33–47.
25. Gregg JA, Callaghan GM, Hayes SC, et al. Improving diabetes self-management through acceptance, mindfulness, and values: a randomized controlled trial. J Consult Clin Psychol 2007;75(2):336–43.

26. Rosenzweig S, Reibel DK, Greeson JM, et al. Mindfulness-based stress reduction is associated with improved glycemic control in type 2 diabetes mellitus: a pilot study. Altern Ther Health Med 2007;13(5):36–8.

27. Kreitzer MJ, Gross CR, Ye X, et al. Longitudinal impact of mindfulness meditation on illness burden in solid-organ transplant recipients. Prog Transplant 2005;15(2): 166–72.

28. Sullivan MJ, Wood L, Terry J, et al. The Support, Education, and Research in Chronic Heart Failure Study (SEARCH): a mindfulness-based psychoeducational intervention improves depression and clinical symptoms in patients with chronic heart failure. Am Heart J 2009;157(1):84–90.

29. Bohlmeijer E, Prenger R, Taal E, et al. The effects of mindfulness-based stress reduction therapy on mental health of adults with a chronic medical disease: a meta-analysis. J Psychosom Res 2010;68(6):539–44.

30. Matousek RH, Dobkin PL, Pruessner J. Cortisol as a marker for improvement in mindfulness-based stress reduction. Complement Ther Clin Pract 2010;16(1): 13–9.

31. Chiesa A, Serretti A. A systematic review of neurobiological and clinical features of mindfulness meditations. Psychol Med 2010;40(8):1239–52.

32. Carmody J, Baer RA, L B Lykins E, et al. An empirical study of the mechanisms of mindfulness in a mindfulness-based stress reduction program. J Clin Psychol 2009;65(6):613–26.

33. Baer RA, Smith GT, Hopkins J, et al. Using self-report assessment methods to explore facets of mindfulness. Assessment 2006;13(1):27–45.

34. Carmody J, Baer RA. Relationships between mindfulness practice and levels of mindfulness, medical and psychological symptoms and well-being in a mindfulness-based stress reduction program. J Behav Med 2008;31(1):23–33.

35. Baer RA, Smith GT, Lykins E, et al. Construct validity of the five facet mindfulness questionnaire in meditating and nonmeditating samples. Assessment 2008;15(3): 329–42.

36. Jha AP, Krompinger J, Baime MJ. Mindfulness training modifies subsystems of attention. Cogn Affect Behav Neurosci 2007;7(2):109–19.

37. Tang YY, Ma Y, Wang J, et al. Short-term meditation training improves attention and self-regulation. Proc Natl Acad Sci U S A 2007;104(43):17152–6.

38. Sanders WA, Lam DH. Ruminative and mindful self-focused processing modes and their impact on problem solving in dysphoric individuals. Behav Res Ther 2010;48(8):747–53.

39. Watkins E, Teasdale JD. Adaptive and maladaptive self-focus in depression. J Affect Disord 2004;82(1):1–8.

40. Linehan MM. Skills training manual for treating borderline personality disorder. New York: Guilford Press; 1993.

41. Moore A, Malinowski P. Meditation, mindfulness and cognitive flexibility. Conscious Cogn 2009;18(1):176–86.

42. Hayes SC, Luoma JB, Bond FW, et al. Acceptance and commitment therapy: model, processes and outcomes. Behav Res Ther 2006;44(1):1–25.

43. Baer RA. Self-focused attention and mechanisms of change in mindfulness-based treatment. Cogn Behav Ther 2009;38(Suppl 1):15–20.

44. Hayes SC. Acceptance and commitment therapy, relational frame theory, and the third wave of behavioral and cognitive therapies. Behav Ther 2004;35(4):639–65.

45. Carmody J, Baer RA. How long does a mindfulness-based stress reduction program need to be? A review of class contact hours and effect sizes for psychological distress. J Clin Psychol 2009;65(6):627–38.

46. Pradhan EK, Baumgarten M, Langenberg P, et al. Effect of mindfulness-based stress reduction in rheumatoid arthritis patients. Arthritis Rheum 2007;57(7): 1134–42.

47. Davidson RJ, Kabat-Zinn J, Schumacher J, et al. Alterations in brain and immune function produced by mindfulness meditation. Psychosom Med 2003;65(4): 564–70.

48. Gross CR, Kreitzer MJ, Russas V, et al. Mindfulness meditation to reduce symptoms after organ transplant: a pilot study. Adv Mind Body Med 2004;20(2):20–9.

49. Rosenzweig S, Greeson JM, Reibel DK, et al. Mindfulness-based stress reduction for chronic pain conditions: variation in treatment outcomes and role of home meditation practice. J Psychosom Res 2010;68(1):29–36.

50. Segal ZV, Williams JM, Teasdale JD. Mindfulness-based cognitive therapy for depression: a new approach to preventing relapse. New York: Guilford Press; 2002.

51. Teasdale JD, Moore RG, Hayhurst H, et al. Metacognitive awareness and prevention of relapse in depression: empirical evidence. J Consult Clin Psychol 2002; 70(2):275–87.

52. Teasdale JD. Cognitive vulnerability to persistent depression. Cogn Emot 1988; 2(3):247–74.

53. Persons JB, Miranda J. Cognitive theories of vulnerability to depression: reconciling negative evidence. Cognit Ther Res 1992;16(4):485–502.

54. Williams M, Teasdale J, Segal Z, et al. The mindful way through depression: freeing yourself from chronic unhappiness. New York: Guilford Press; 2007.

55. Linehan MM, Armstrong HE, Suarez A, et al. Cognitive-behavioral treatment of chronically parasuicidal borderline patients. Arch Gen Psychiatry 1991;48(12): 1060–4.

56. Fitzcharles MA, Shir Y. New concepts in rheumatic pain. Rheum Dis Clin North Am 2008;34(2):267–83.

57. Montecucco C, Cavagna L, Caporali R. Pain and rheumatology: an overview of the problem. European Journal of Pain Supplements 2009;3(2):105–9.

58. Reginster JY, Khaltaev NG. Introduction and WHO perspective on the global burden of musculoskeletal conditions. Rheumatology (Oxford) 2002;41(Supp 1): 1–2.

59. Fitzcharles MA, Almahrezi A, Shir Y. Pain: understanding and challenges for the rheumatologist. Arthritis Rheum 2005;52(12):3685–92.

60. Borenstein D. The role of the rheumatologist in managing pain therapy. Nat Rev Rheumatol 2010;6(4):227–31.

61. Integration of behavioral and relaxation approaches into the treatment of chronic pain and insomnia. NIH Technology Assessment Panel on Integration of Behavioral and Relaxation Approaches into the Treatment of Chronic Pain and Insomnia. JAMA 1996;276(4):313–8.

62. Wolsko PM, Eisenberg DM, Davis RB, et al. Use of mind-body medical therapies. J Gen Intern Med 2004;19(1):43–50.

63. Astin JA, Beckner W, Soeken K, et al. Psychological interventions for rheumatoid arthritis: a meta-analysis of randomized controlled trials. Arthritis Rheum 2002; 47(3):291–302.

64. Dixon KE, Keefe FJ, Scipio CD, et al. Psychological interventions for arthritis pain management in adults: a meta-analysis. Health Psychol 2007;26(3):241–50.

65. McCracken LM. Behavioral constituents of chronic pain acceptance: results from factor analysis of the chronic pain acceptance questionnaire. J Back Musculoskelet Rehabil 1999;13(2):93–100.

66. Brown CA, Jones AK. Meditation experience predicts less negative appraisal of pain: electrophysiological evidence for the involvement of anticipatory neural responses. Pain 2010;150(3):428–38.
67. McCracken LM, Gauntlett-Gilbert J, Vowles KE. The role of mindfulness in a contextual cognitive-behavioral analysis of chronic pain-related suffering and disability. Pain 2007;131(1–2):63–9.
68. Schutze R, Rees C, Preece M, et al. Low mindfulness predicts pain catastrophizing in a fear-avoidance model of chronic pain. Pain 2010;148(1):120–7.
69. Zautra AJ, Davis MC, Reich JW, et al. Comparison of cognitive behavioral and mindfulness meditation interventions on adaptation to rheumatoid arthritis for patients with and without history of recurrent depression. J Consult Clin Psychol 2008;76(3):408–21.
70. Morone NE, Greco CM, Weiner DK. Mindfulness meditation for the treatment of chronic low back pain in older adults: a randomized controlled pilot study. Pain 2008;134(3):310–9.
71. Morone NE, Rollman BL, Moore CG, et al. A mind-body program for older adults with chronic low back pain: results of a pilot study. Pain Med 2009;10(8):1395–407.
72. Goldenberg DL, Kaplan KH, Nadeau MG, et al. A controlled study of a stress-reduction, cognitive-behavioral treatment program in fibromyalgia. J Muscoskel Pain 1994;2(2):53–66.
73. Grossman P, Tiefenthaler-Gilmer U, Raysz A, et al. Mindfulness training as an intervention for fibromyalgia: evidence of postintervention and 3-year follow-up benefits in well-being. Psychother Psychosom 2007;76(4):226–33.
74. Astin JA, Berman BM, Bausell B, et al. The efficacy of mindfulness meditation plus Qigong movement therapy in the treatment of fibromyalgia: a randomized controlled trial. J Rheumatol 2003;30(10):2257–62.
75. Coelho HF, Canter PH, Ernst E. Mindfulness-based cognitive therapy: evaluating current evidence and informing future research. J Consult Clin Psychol 2007;75(6):1000–5.
76. Godfrin KA, van Heeringen C. The effects of mindfulness-based cognitive therapy on recurrence of depressive episodes, mental health and quality of life: a randomized controlled study. Behav Res Ther 2010;48(8):738–46.
77. Williams JM, Alatiq Y, Crane C, et al. Mindfulness-based cognitive therapy (MBCT) in bipolar disorder: preliminary evaluation of immediate effects on between-episode functioning. J Affect Disord 2008;107(1–3):275–9.
78. Sephton SE, Salmon P, Weissbecker I, et al. Mindfulness meditation alleviates depressive symptoms in women with fibromyalgia: results of a randomized clinical trial. Arthritis Rheum 2007;57(1):77–85.
79. Weissbecker I, Salmon P, Studts JL, et al. Mindfulness-based stress reduction and sense of coherence among women with fibromyalgia. J Clin Psychol Med Settings 2002;9(4):297–307.
80. Finucane A, Mercer SW. An exploratory mixed methods study of the acceptability and effectiveness of mindfulness-based cognitive therapy for patients with active depression and anxiety in primary care. BMC Psychiatry 2006;6:14.
81. Eisendrath SJ, Delucchi K, Bitner R, et al. Mindfulness-based cognitive therapy for treatment-resistant depression: a pilot study. Psychother Psychosom 2008;77(5):319–20.
82. Glaser R, Kiecolt-Glaser JK. Stress-induced immune dysfunction: implications for health. Nat Rev Immunol 2005;5(3):243–51.

83. Carlson LE, Speca M, Faris P, et al. One year pre-post intervention follow-up of psychological, immune, endocrine and blood pressure outcomes of mindfulness-based stress reduction (MBSR) in breast and prostate cancer outpatients. Brain Behav Immun 2007;21(8):1038–49.

84. Robinson FP, Mathews HL, Witek-Janusek L. Psycho-endocrine-immune response to mindfulness-based stress reduction in individuals infected with the human immunodeficiency virus: a quasiexperimental study. J Altern Complement Med 2003;9(5):683–94.

85. Witek-Janusek L, Albuquerque K, Chroniak KR, et al. Effect of mindfulness based stress reduction on immune function, quality of life and coping in women newly diagnosed with early stage breast cancer. Brain Behav Immun 2008;22(6): 969–81.

86. Fang CY, Reibel DK, Longacre ML, et al. Enhanced psychosocial well-being following participation in a mindfulness-based stress reduction program is associated with increased natural killer cell activity. J Altern Complement Med 2010; 16(5):531–8.

87. Ospina MB, Bond K, Karkhaneh M, et al. Meditation practices for health: state of the research. Evid Rep Technol Assess (Full Rep) 2007;155:1–263.

Fish Oil in Rheumatic Diseases

Samir Bhangle, MD, Sharon L. Kolasinski, MD*

KEYWORDS

- Fish oil • Polyunsaturated fatty acids • Arachidonic acid
- Anti-inflammatory

In current practice, dietary interventions and over-the-counter dietary supplements, including fish oil, vitamins, and others, comprise a significant proportion of alternate therapy use. In spite of substantial data and compelling evidence about the efficacy of using fish oil in the treatment of rheumatoid arthritis (RA) and possible use in other inflammatory diseases, questions remain regarding the mechanism of action, correct dosage, and the potential for possible side effects and medication interactions. The aim of this article is to clarify the appropriate place for the use of fish oil in rheumatologic practice amid the complexities of modern management.

The first data to suggest the possible antiinflammatory effects of omega-3 (n-3) fatty acids were derived from the epidemiologic studies of the Greenland Eskimos by Kronmann and Green[1] in 1980. The lower prevalence of diseases such as acute myocardial infarction, diabetes mellitus, thyrotoxicosis, bronchial asthma, multiple sclerosis, and psoriasis, which are increasingly thought to have some inflammatory component, in Greenland Eskimos compared with that in the inhabitants of Western countries has been postulated to be due to their diet rich in seafood containing high amounts of long-chain polyunsaturated fatty acids (PUFAs). Since this early report, there has been a large amount of biochemical and clinical data and many studies to support the use of PUFAs in a variety of chronic conditions in which inflammation is thought to play a central role in pathogenesis.

CHEMISTRY OF DIETARY FATTY ACIDS

There are 3 major classes of fatty acids: saturated fatty acids (no double bonds); monounsaturated fatty acids (single double bond); and PUFAs ($\geq$2 double bonds). The PUFAs are subclassified into n-3 or n-6 PUFAs according to the site of the double bond (at the third or the sixth position) proximal to the methyl terminus. Enzymes required to introduce the double bonds into the n-3 and n-6 positions are not present in mammals, and therefore, these fatty acids must be obtained from the diet and are accordingly termed as essential fatty acids. The n-3 fatty acids can be derived from

Division of Rheumatology, University of Pennsylvania School of Medicine, 8 Penn Tower, 34th Street and Civic Center Boulevard, PA 19104, USA
* Corresponding author.
E-mail address: Sharon.Kolasinski@uphs.upenn.edu

Rheum Dis Clin N Am 37 (2011) 77–84
doi:10.1016/j.rdc.2010.11.003
0889-857X/11/$ – see front matter © 2011 Elsevier Inc. All rights reserved.

fish and plant sources, but with certain fundamental differences. The fish-derived n-3 fatty acids, eicosapentaenoic acid (EPA) and docosahexaenoic acid (DHA), have longer carbon chains and are more unsaturated than the plant-derived n-3 fatty acids, alpha-linolenic acid (ALA), and stearidonic acid.

In a typical Western diet, far more n-6 fat is consumed than n-3 fat[2] mainly because of the abundance of linoleic acid (LA) in soybean, safflower, sunflower, and corn oils, which are readily available for food preparation and are present in many processed foods. The chemical similarity between n-3 and n-6 PUFAs leads to competitive inhibition of metabolism of n-3 by n-6 fatty acids and vice versa. Because LA is the n-6 homolog of ALA, it can decrease metabolism of vegetable oil–derived ALA to EPA and also decrease the level of tissue EPA plus DHA that has arisen from dietary EPA plus DHA. Thus, the relatively high LA intake in the American diet presents an important practical barrier to dietary strategies aimed at elevating tissue levels of EPA plus DHA and exerting their beneficial effects.[3]

MECHANISM OF ACTION OF N-3 FATTY ACIDS

A number of antiinflammatory mechanisms have been postulated to account for the beneficial effects of fish oil. These include alteration of arachidonic acid (AA) pathway products favoring antiinflammatory mediators and disruption of adhesion molecule activity.

Both EPA and DHA are homologous to AA. They competitively inhibit the oxidation of AA by cyclooxygenase (COX) to n-6 prostaglandins (PGs). They also inhibit the conversion of AA to leukotrienes (LTs) via 5-lipoxygenase (LOX) enzymes. These PGs and LTs are collectively referred to as eicosanoids (C20 oxylipids). The n-6 eicosanoids PGE2, thromboxane A2 (TXA2), and leukotriene B4 (LTB4) are all proinflammatory. PGE2 causes vasodilatation, increased vascular permeability, and hyperalgesia.[4,5] TXA2 promotes synthesis of inflammatory cytokines, interleukin (IL) 1 beta, and tumor necrosis factor α (TNF-α) by mononuclear phagocytes.[6] LTB4 is a neutrophil chemoattractant and activator.[1] In addition to reducing the production of n-6 eicosanoids, dietary fish oil has also been shown to inhibit TNF-α and IL-1 synthesis in healthy human beings and patients with RA.[7–10] With the inhibition of formation of these proinflammatory cytokines by EPA and DHA, the net result is reduction in all the cardinal signs of inflammation, such as pain, warmth, redness, swelling, and loss of function.

Interestingly, it is not simply the downregulation of proinflammatory cytokines that contributes to this antiinflammatory effect. In addition, antiinflammatory cytokines are also increased. EPA and DHA are substrates for antiinflammatory eicosanoid formation. DHA can be converted via 15-LOX to 17(S)- and 17(R)-hydroxyl derivatives to a compound called resolvin D1. Resolvin production via the COX-2 pathway also happens when aspirin is given. Resolvins have antiinflammatory effects in the murine peritonitis model by downregulating leukocyte recruitment and stimulating macrophage removal of apoptotic cells.[11,12]

Beyond effects on cytokine levels, the n-3 fatty acids, in vitro and ex vivo, have been shown to decrease the expression of adhesion molecules, intercellular adhesion molecule (ICAM) 1, and leukocyte function–associated antigen (LFA) 1.[13–15] ICAM-1 and LFA-1 have been implicated in the migration of leukocytes in the inflamed synovium in laboratory rodents,[16] and ICAM-1 blockade has been shown to reduce disease activity in RA.[17]

In RA and other inflammatory joint diseases, chronic joint inflammation causes cartilage destruction by the various matrix metalloproteinases (MMPs), which serve as the ultimate effector molecules. N-3 fatty acid supplementation abolishes the expression of messenger RNA (mRNA) for MMP-13 and MMP-3 in human cartilage and reduction of proteoglycan degradation as seen in IL-1 stimulated bovine chondrocytes.[18,19] Thus, the n-3 fatty acids exert a vast array of antiinflammatory effects via a number of different mechanisms.

CLINICAL STUDIES OF FISH OIL IN RA

In addition to the pharmacologic and laboratory evidence, there have been 14 double-blind, randomized controlled trials reporting the clinical outcomes and the beneficial effects of fish oil in RA.[20] Almost all the 14 trials have been undertaken in patients with late disease, with mean duration of more than 10 years.[21] The outcomes measured in these trials often included reduction in the tender joints and duration of morning stiffness after starting fish oil treatment. These analyses concluded that fish oil provided a reduction in the number of tender joints and duration of the morning stiffness. These benefits in RA have also been supported by meta-analysis and mega-analysis of outcomes after 12 weeks of fish oil supplementation.[22] Goldberg and Katz[23] conducted a meta-analysis of 17 randomized control trials that included assessment of the analgesic effects of n-3 fatty acid supplementation in patients with RA or joint pain secondary to inflammatory bowel disease. It concluded that fish oil decreased the intensity of joint pain, duration of morning stiffness, number of tender and swollen joints, and the use of nonsteroidal antiinflammatory drugs (NSAIDs). Furthermore, in 2 studies, some subjects who ingested fish oil were able to sustain a lower NSAID dose even after fish oil supplements were discontinued.[24–28] The beneficial antiinflammatory effects of fish oil in RA are generally delayed by up to 12 weeks after they are started. There is also a dose response for time of onset of symptomatic benefits, with reduction in latency seen with higher doses of fish oil.[27,29] Clinical benefits have been observed to last for up to 6 weeks after discontinuing therapy.[29] However, most of the studies of fish oil in RA have involved relatively a small number of subjects (N = 16–67). Also, all the clinical trials to date in RA have been in patients with a long-standing disease. The role of fish oil in early disease is not well explored. Trials investigating long-term outcomes of n-3 fatty acid supplementation in a setting where multiple and changing medications are used are also lacking.

OTHER INFLAMMATORY DISEASES

Consumption of n-3 PUFAs suppresses inflammatory processes that would be extended to management and trials of other inflammatory diseases. Several recent trials have provided evidence that n-3 PUFA supplementation could be useful in treatment of human immunoglobulin A (IgA) nephropathy and lupus nephritis, whereas others suggest such supplementation might be without benefit.[30,31] Duffy and colleagues[32] in their double-blind, double placebo controlled factorial trial concluded that dietary supplementation with fish oil may be beneficial in modifying symptomatic disease activity in patients with systemic lupus erythematosus (SLE). The reported favorable influence of fish oil on relapse rates in Crohn disease is also worth noting.[33] N-3 fatty acids lower plasma triglyceride levels, particularly in persons with hypertriglyceridemia, by inhibiting the synthesis of very-low-density lipoprotein cholesterol and triglycerides in the liver.[34]

They have been reported to have a dose-response blood pressure–lowering effect in patients with hypertension and with little or no effect in patients with normal blood pressure.[35] N-3 fatty acids have been shown in epidemiologic and clinical trials to reduce the incidence of cerebrovascular disease. Evidence from prospective secondary prevention studies suggest that EPA plus DHA consumption ranging from 0.5 to 1.8 g/d (either as fatty fish or supplementation) significantly reduces subsequent cardiac and all-cause mortality.[36] One study showed increased regression and decreased progression of coronary lesions in patients taking 1.5 g/d of fish oil for 2 years, as assessed by angiography.[37]

Thus, some have suggested that fish oil could have a cardioprotective role, which warrants further investigations.

OSTEOARTHRITIS

Continuing interest has surrounded the use of fish oil supplementation in the therapy of osteoarthritis (OA), despite the fact that OA is generally thought of as a noninflammatory condition. In diverse locations around the world, 5% to 40% of subjects surveyed in epidemiologic studies have responded that they have used fish oil for treatment of OA.[38,39] Early studies were not encouraging. A group of 86 subjects were given either 10 mL of cod liver oil or an equal volume of olive oil daily for 24 weeks.[40] The 2 groups did not differ significantly in their NSAID dose or in their physician or patient visual analog scores for pain and for disability at the end of the trial. Nonetheless, subsequent laboratory studies established effects of n-3 PUFAs that were relevant to OA pathophysiology. Human OA cartilage explanted at the time of total knee replacement was exposed for 24 hours to n-3 PUFAs, n-6 PUFAs, or a mixture of monounsaturated and saturated fatty acids (oleate and palmitate).[18] Exposure to n-3 PUFAs, but not other fatty acids, reduced, in a dose-dependent manner, the endogenous and IL-1–induced release of proteoglycan metabolites from the articular cartilage explants and also abolished endogenous aggrecanase and collagenase proteolytic activities as well as expression of mRNA for ADAMTS-4, MMP-13, and MMP-3 and mRNA for proinflammatory mediators (COX-2, 5-LOX, 5- LOX–activating protein, TNF-α, IL-1). Tissue inhibitor of metalloproteinase levels was unaffected. These results have recently been replicated in bovine chondrocyte cultures.[41]

Recent work has focused on a more macroscopic examination of the influence of fatty acid composition of the diet on bone health. Investigators prospectively followed 297 subjects within the Melbourne Collaborative Cohort Study who had no history ofOA.[42] They collected dietary and demographic data at baseline between 1990 and 1994 and performed magnetic resonance imaging of the knees on the same individuals during 2003 and 2004. The researchers found that ingestion of total and n-6 PUFAs were associated with the presence of bone marrow lesions (BMLs) in univariate analysis and after adjustment for calorie intake, age, gender, and body mass index. Intake of monounsaturated fatty acids was positively associated with the presence of BMLs in multivariate analysis. On the other hand, n-3 PUFAs were not associated with these predictors of knee pain and cartilage loss in OA. A number of veterinary studies have suggested improvements in mobility with fish oil supplementation,[43] but conclusive evidence of a clinically significant effect of fish oil in OA remains to be seen.

DOSE AND ROUTE OF ADMINISTRATION OF N-3 FATTY ACIDS

Symptomatic benefits have been reported with doses between 2.6 and 7.1 g/d, with no effect seen at 1 g/d. Such high doses can be realistically achieved only with fish oil, but the cost of treatment can substantially exceed that of many other medications. Cost savings accrue to those using the two-glass technique and unencapsulated fish oil. This technique involves floating 10 to 15 mL of fish oil on about 30 mL of fruit or vegetable juice in a small glass. This is placed in the mouth to allow the contents to be swallowed without contacting the lips, thereby avoiding the fish oil taste.

Immediately after swallowing, a further 40 mL or so of juice is taken from a separate glass to rinse the mouth. If taken before a solid meal without additional fluid, a repeating dose can also be avoided. Lying on the left side for 10 minutes immediately after ingestion to drain the stomach contents into the duodenum is another strategy for avoiding "repeating" fish oil taste.[21] By using this method, there have been approximately 6- and 2-fold increases in EPA and DHA levels, respectively and a decrease in AA levels by 30% to 40%.[44,45] Of note, vegetable oils containing the n-3 fatty acid, ALA, can also elevate EPA albeit much less effectively. However, vegetable oils containing the n-6 fatty acid, LA, decrease tissue EPA arising from dietary EPA or dietary ALA. Thus, tissue levels of antiinflammatory n-3 fatty acids, EPA plus DHA can be most effectively increased by a combination of all of the following: fish oil supplements, fish meals, n-3–containing vegetable oils (such as canola and flaxseed oils), and avoidance of n-6–containing vegetable oils (such as peanut, cottonseed, sunflower, and soybean oils) by substituting monounsaturated vegetable oils (such as olive and canola oils).[3]

INTERACTIONS AND ADVERSE EFFECTS

Although generally considered safe, fish oil may have some unwanted side effects. The most common side effects of n-3 fatty acids are a fishy aftertaste and gastrointestinal disturbances, both of which seem to be dose dependent.[36] In 2 studies, gastrointestinal upset was reported in 4.9% and 8% of patients taking 0.85 and 6.9 g/d of n-3 fatty acids, respectively.[46] High doses of fish oil may increase levels of low-density lipoprotein cholesterol, the clinical relevance of which remains uncertain.[34,47] Although n-3 fatty acids exert a dose-related effect on bleeding time, there have been no documented cases of abnormal bleeding caused by fish oil supplementation, even at high doses and in combination with other anticoagulant medications.[48] The initial concerns that fish oil can worsen hyperglycemia seem to be unfounded after a recent meta-analysis concluded that fish oil supplements in the range of 3 to 18 g/d had no statistically significant effect on glycemic control and fasting blood glucose and hemoglobin A1C levels.[49] The Food and Drug Administration has categorized EPA and DHA n-3 fatty acids as dietary supplements, as up to 3 g/d of their consumption.[50,51] Furthermore, fish oil supplements are essentially free of mercury and other contaminants that may be present in fish, thus can be safely consumed by all.[34] Thus, fish oil supplements for the most part are relatively safe in doses needed to exert their antiinflammatory effects.

SUMMARY

Considerable high-quality evidence suggests that there are clinically beneficial effects of dietary fish oil in inflammatory and cardiovascular diseases. Because of the inhibition of proinflammatory cytokines, such as IL-1β and TNF-α, as well as other mechanisms, fish oil reduces inflammation. Fish oil can reduce the use of NSAIDs as seen in meta-analyses in patients with RA, thus conferring additional cardiovascular benefits and preventing the gastrointestinal adverse effects associated with NSAID use. Symptomatic benefits are seen with doses between 2.6 to 7.1 g/d. The beneficial antiinflammatory effects of fish oil in RA are generally delayed by up to 12 weeks after their commencement and can be seen up to 6 weeks after their discontinuation. They are relatively free of side effects except for the fishy aftertaste and some gastrointestinal disturbances. Their purported beneficial effects in IgA nephropathy, SLE, lupus nephritis, Crohn disease, and OA warrant further studies.

REFERENCES

1. Kronmann N, Green A. Epidemiological studies in the Upernavik district, Greenland: incidence of some chronic diseases 1950–1974. Acta Med Scand 1980;208:401–6.
2. Simopoulos AP. N-3 fatty acids in health and disease and in growth and development. Am J Clin Nutr 1991;54:438–63.
3. Proudman SM, Cleland LG, James MJ. Dietary omega-3 fats for the treatment of inflammatory joint disease: efficacy and utility. Rheum Dis Clin North Am 2008;34:469–79.
4. Salmmon JA, Higgs GA. Prostaglandins and leukotrienes as inflammatory mediators. Br Med Bull 1987;43:285–96.
5. Samuelsson B. Leukotrienes: mediators of immediate hypersensitivity reactions and inflammation. Science 1983;220:568–75.
6. Caughey GE, Pouliot M, Cleland LG, et al. Regulation of tumor necrosis factor-alpha and IL-1 beta synthesis by thromboxane A2 in non-adherent human monocytes. J Immunol 1997;158:351–8.
7. Mantzioris E, Cleland LG, Gibson RA, et al. Biochemical effects of a diet containing foods enriched with n-3 fatty acids. Am J Clin Nutr 2000;72:42–8.
8. Caughey GE, mantzoris E, Gibson RA, et al. The effect on human tumor necrosis factor alpha and interleukin-1 beta of diets enriched in n-3 fatty acids from vegetable oil or fish oil. Am J Clin Nutr 1996;63:116–22.
9. Endres S, Ghorbani R, Kelley VE, et al. The effect of dietary supplementation with n-3 polyunsaturated fatty acids on the synthesis of interleukin-1 and tumor necrosis factor by mononuclear cells. N Engl J Med 1989;320:265–71.
10. Meydani SN, Endres S, Woods MM, et al. Oral (n-3) fatty acid supplementation suppresses cytokine production and lymphocyte proliferation: comparison between young and older women. J Nutr 1991;121:547–55.
11. Sun YP, Oh SF, Gronert K, et al. Resolvin D1 and its aspirin-triggered 17 R epimer: stereoisomer assignments, anti-inflammatory properties, and enzymic inactivation. J Biol Chem 2007;282:9323–34.
12. Serhan CN, Hong S, Gronert K, et al. Resolvins: a family of bioactive products of omega-3 fatty acid transformation circuits initiated by aspirin treatment that counter proinflammation signals. J Exp Med 2002;196:1025–37.
13. Hughes DA, Southon S, Pinder A. (n-3) Polyunsaturated fatty acids modulate the expression of functionally associated molecules on human monocytes in vitro. J Nutr 1996;126:603–10.
14. Hughes DA, Pinder AC. (n-3) Polyunsaturated fatty acids inhibit the antigen-presenting function of human monocytes. Am J Clin Nutr 2000;71:357S–60S.
15. Hughes DA, Pinder AC, Piper Z, et al. Fish oil supplementation inhibits the expression of major histocompatibility complex class II molecules and adhesion molecules on human monocytes. Am J Clin Nutr 1996;63:267–72.
16. Liao H-X, Haynes BF. Role of adhesion molecules in the pathogenesis of rheumatoid arthritis. Rheum Dis Clin North Am 1995;21:715–40.
17. Kavanagh AF, Davis LS, Nichols L, et al. Treatment of rheumatoid arthritis with a monoclonal antibody to intercellular adhesion molecule 1. Arthritis Rheum 1994;37:992–9.
18. Curtis C, Rees S, Little C, et al. Pathological indicators of degradation and inflammation in human osteoarthritis cartilage are abrogated by exposure to n-3 fatty acids. Arthritis Rheum 2002;46:1544–53.
19. Curtis C, Hughes C, Flannery C, et al. n-3 fatty acids specifically modulate catabolic factors involved in articular cartilage degradation. J Biol Chem 2000;275: 721–4.

20. Stamp L, James M, Cleland L. Diet and rheumatoid arthritis: a review of the literature. Semin Arthritis Rheum 2005;35:77–94.
21. Cleland LG, James JM, Proudman SM. The role of fish oils in the treatment of rheumatoid arthritis. Drugs 2003;9:845–53.
22. Fortin PR, Lew RA, Liang MH, et al. Validation of a meta-analysis: the effects of fish oil in rheumatoid arthritis. J Clin Epidemiol 1995;48:1379–90.
23. Goldberg RJ, Katz J. A meta-analysis of the analgesic effects of omega-3 polyunsaturated fatty acid supplementation for inflammatory joint pain. Pain 2007; 129:210–23.
24. Skoldstam L, Borjesson O, Kjallman A, et al. Effects of six months of fish oil supplementation in stable rheumatoid arthritis. A double blind, controlled study. Scand J Rheumatol 1992;21:178–85.
25. Lau CS, Morley KD, Belch JJ. Effects of fish oil supplementation on non-steroidal anti-inflammatory drug requirement in patients with mild rheumatoid arthritis-a double blind placebo controlled study. Br J Rheumatol 1993;32:982–9.
26. Geusens P, Wouters C, Nijs J, et al. Long term effect of omega-3 fatty acid supplementation in active rheumatoid arthritis. Arthritis Rheum 1994;37:824–9.
27. Kremer JM, Lawrence DA, Petrillo GF, et al. Effects of high-dose fish oil on rheumatoid arthritis after stopping nonsteroidal anti-inflammatory drugs. Arthritis Rheum 1995;38:1107–14.
28. Kjeldsen-Kragh J, Lund JA, Riise T, et al. Dietary omega-3 fatty acid supplementation and naproxen treatment in patients with rheumatoid arthritis. J Rheumatol 1992;19:1531–6.
29. Kremer JM, Lawrence DA, Jubiz W, et al. Dietary fish oil and olive oil supplementation in patients with rheumatoid arthritis. Arthritis Rheum 1990;33:810–9.
30. Pestka JJ. n-3 polyunsaturated fatty acids and autoimmune-mediated glomerulonephritis. Prostaglandins Leukot Essent Fatty Acids 2010;82(4–6):251–8.
31. Donadio JV. The emerging role of omega-3 polyunsaturated fatty acids in the management of patients with IgA nephropathy. J Ren Nutr 2001;11:122–8.
32. Duffy EM, Meenagh GK, McMillan SA, et al. The clinical effect of dietary supplementation with omega-3 fish oils and/or copper in systemic lupus erythematosus. J Rheumatol 2004;8:1551–6.
33. Belluzzi A, Brignola C, Campieri M, et al. Effect of an enteric-coated fish-oil preparation on relapses on crohn's disease. N Engl J Med 1996;334:1557–60.
34. Harris WS, Ginsberg SN, Arunakul N, et al. Safety and efficacy of Omacor in severe hypertriglyceridemia. J Cardiovasc Risk 1997;4:385–91.
35. Howe PR. Dietary fats and hypertension. Focus on fish oil. Ann N Y Acad Sci 1997;827:339–52.
36. Kris-Etherton PM, Harris WS, Appel LJ. Fish consumption, fish oil, omega-3 fatty acids, and cardiovascular disease. Circulation 2002;106:2747–57.
37. Von Schacky C, Angerer P, Kothny W, et al. The effect of dietary omega-3 fatty acids on coronary atherosclerosis. A randomized, double blind, placebo controlled trial. Ann Intern Med 1999;130:554–62.
38. Zochling J, March LM, Lapsley H, et al. Use of complementary medicines for osteoarthritis—a prospective study. Ann Rheum Dis 2004;63:549–54.
39. Jordan KM, Sawyer S, Coakley P, et al. The use of conventional and complementary treatments for knee osteoarthritis in the community. Rheumatology 2004;43:381–4.
40. Stammers T, Sibbald B, Freeling P. Efficacy of cod liver oil as an adjunct to non-steroidal anti-inflammatory drug treatment in the management of osteoarthritis in general. Ann Rheum Dis 1992;51:128–9.

41. Zainal Z, Longman AJ, Hurst S, et al. Relative efficacies of omega-3 polyunsaturated fatty acids in reducing expression of key proteins in a model system for studying osteoarthritis. Osteoarthritis Cartilage 2009;17:896–905.

42. Wnag Y, Wluka AE, Hodge AM, et al. Effect of fatty acids on bone marrow lesions and knee cartilage in healthy middle-aged subjects without clinical knee osteoarthritis. Osteoarthritis Cartilage 2008;16:579–83.

43. Roush JK, Cross AR, Renberg WC, et al. Evaluation of the effects of dietary supplementation with fish oil omega-3 fatty acids on weight bearing in dogs with osteoarthritis. J Am Vet Med Assoc 2010;236(1):67–73.

44. Cleland LG, Proudman SM, Hall C, et al. A biomarker of n-3 compliance in patients taking fish oil for rheumatoid arthritis. Lipids 2003;38:419–24.

45. Cleland LG, Caughey GE, James MJ, et al. Reduction of cardiovascular risk factors with longterm fish oil treatment in early rheumatoid arthritis. J Rheumatol 2006;33:1973–9.

46. Gruppo Italiano per lo Studio della Sopravvivenza nell' Infarto miocardico. Dietary supplementation with n-3 polyunsaturated fatty acids and vitamin E after myocardial infarction: results of the GISSI-Prevenzione trial. Lancet 1999;354:447–55.

47. Harris WS. N-3 fatty acids and serum lipoproteins: human studies. Am J Clin Nutr 1997;65:1645S–54S.

48. Eritsland J, Arnesen H, Gronseth K, et al. Effect of dietary supplementation with n-3 fatty acids on coronary artery bypass graft patency. Am J Cardiol 1996;77:31–6.

49. Montori V, Farmer A, Wollan P, et al. Fish oil supplementation in type 2 diabetes: a quantitative systematic review. Diabetes Care 2000;23:1217–8.

50. Department of Health and Human Services. US Food and Drug Administration. Substances affirmed as generally recognized as safe: menhaden oil. Fed Regist 1997;62:30751–7.

51. Office of Nutritional Products. Labeling, and dietary supplements, center for food safety and applied nutrition. US Food and Drug Administration; 2002. Available at: http://www.fda.gov/AboutFDA/CentersOffices/OrganizationCharts/ucm135675.htm. Accessed November 8, 2010.

The State of Research on Complementary and Alternative Medicine in Pediatric Rheumatology

Karine Toupin April, OT, PhD[a,b,*], Rishma Walji, ND, PhD[c]

KEYWORDS

- Pediatric rheumatology • Juvenile idiopathic arthritis
- Complementary and alternative medicine

Because of the growing interest in unconventional therapies, health care providers caring for children are increasingly asked to recommend relevant, safe, cost-effective, and age-appropriate treatments regardless of whether or not they are considered to be conventional medicine. Interest in unconventional medicine, also called complementary and alternative medicine (CAM), among families and health care providers is increasing.[1] Between 1994 and 2003, pediatric CAM use increased from 10% to 35%, depending on the study.[2] Estimates vary depending on the country (approximately 2% of children in the United States, 11% in Canada, 18% in the United Kingdom, and 31% in Australia)[3–6] but even more so on the type of patient population surveyed. For instance, children with chronic illnesses[7] as well as adolescents (with or without chronic disease) are frequent users (57% use in the past year for the former and 79% lifetime use for the latter).[8]

The authors have nothing to disclose.

CAM research being conducted by the authors was funded by grants from the Canadian Institutes of Health Research, the Sick Kids Foundation, the Canadian Arthritis Network, and the Arthritis Society of Canada. K.T.A. was supported by a postdoctoral fellowship award from the Canadian Arthritis Network and the Canadian Institutes of Health Research. R.W. was supported by a postdoctoral fellowship award from the Canadian Health Services Research Foundation.

[a] Department of Epidemiology and Community Medicine, University of Ottawa, Room 3105451 Smyth Road, Ottawa, ON K1H 8M5, Canada

[b] Institute of Population Health, University of Ottawa, 1 Stewart Street, Room 201, Ottawa, ON K1N 6N5, Canada

[c] Department of Health, Aging and Society, McMaster University, Kenneth Taylor Hall, Room 240, 1280 Main Street West, Hamilton, ON L8S 4M4, Canada

* Corresponding author. Department of Epidemiology and Community Medicine, University of Ottawa, Room 3105451 Smyth Road, Ottawa, ON K1H 8M5, Canada.
E-mail address: ktoupina@uottawa.ca

Rheum Dis Clin N Am 37 (2011) 85–94
doi:10.1016/j.rdc.2010.11.011
0889-857X/11/$ – see front matter © 2011 Elsevier Inc. All rights reserved.

Not surprisingly, children and youth with juvenile idiopathic arthritis (JIA) and other pediatric rheumatology conditions also use these treatments regularly.[9–14] Despite their high use and good reported effectiveness by parents, little is known about the efficacy of unconventional therapies in patients with JIA. Parents also seem to be reluctant to disclose its use to their treating physicians,[12] and health care providers do not always inquire about the use of therapies in routine clinical care.[15] This lack of awareness could be problematic because using these therapies in combination with conventional care may be beneficial but may also lead to a higher burden of care or diminished efficacy of medications.[16] Adverse effects are also possible, and pharmacologic interactions exist with prescribed medication.[17]

This article discusses the use of CAM in pediatric rheumatology as well as the characteristics and perceptions of parents who use these treatments for their child. Data about the efficacy and safety of the most commonly used types of CAM in addition to the potential challenges and avenues for future research in this field are also presented.

WHAT IS CAM

According to the National Center for Complementary and Alternative Medicine (NCCAM), a part of the National Institutes of Health in the United States, complementary medicine includes many types of therapies and products that are not considered to be a part of conventional medicine. The NCCAM divides complementary medicine into 5 domains: (1) alternative medical systems (eg, homeopathy, naturopathy, traditional Chinese medicine), (2) mind-body interventions (eg, hypnosis, biofeedback), (3) biologically based therapies (eg, herbal supplements, aromatherapy), (4) manipulative and body-based methods (eg, chiropractic, massage therapy), and (5) energy therapies (eg, therapeutic touch).[18] However, there is no consensus on the definition of complementary medicine and on the types of therapies or products that should be considered as such. For now, the best way to deal with the many definitions is to make sure that researchers and clinicians explain clearly what they mean by CAM when they gather the data. In this article, the term CAM is used because it is inclusive of many different types of therapies, products, and health systems and has been used in other publications.[14,19] Also, the NCCAM classification has been referred to here.

CHARACTERISTICS OF USERS
Use of CAM

To date, there have been 5 studies documenting the use of CAM in children with JIA, arthralgia, connective tissue disease (systemic lupus erythematosus, dermatomyositis, scleroderma, or vasculitis), or other pediatric conditions treated by pediatric rheumatologists (including fibromyalgia and rare diagnoses such as sarcoidosis).[9–14,19] Of these studies, 4 were cross-sectional and 1 described the use of CAM during a 1-year period. According to studies in pediatric rheumatology, the percentage of CAM use ranges between 34% and 92%. In the longitudinal study, use of CAM ranged between 10% and 24% for the various 3-month intervals, and 51% of participants had used CAM in the past to treat their JIA symptoms.[14] Among these participants, 36% used CAM for more than a 3-month interval.[14]

Types of CAM Used

According to the study by Southwood and colleagues[9] conducted in 1990[9] surveying 53 children with JIA from Canada (n = 18), New Zealand (n = 4), and Australia (n = 31) attending a summer camp, 70% of participants reported having used unconventional therapies. The most common therapies were copper bracelets, diet modifications, natural health products (NHPs), and chiropractic. High CAM use could be explained in part by the high disease severity of these children. In 1999, a study conducted by Hagen and colleagues[10] on 141 children attending an outpatient rheumatology clinic and diagnosed with one of arthritis, connective tissue disease (systemic lupus erythematosus, dermatomyositis, scleroderma, or vasculitis), or other pediatric conditions (including fibromyalgia, rare diagnoses such as sarcoidosis, and those illnesses not yet diagnosed) at a tertiary care children's hospital, 64% of the children used at least one type of CAM in the past year and half of them, more than one type. The most used interventions were vitamins, minerals, relaxation techniques, chiropractic, and homeopathy. High CAM use could be explained by the emphasis given to nutritional supplements in the survey. In fact, the use was lower (51.8%) when vitamins and minerals were excluded. Zebracki and colleagues[12] also showed a high level of CAM use in 36 Latin American children with JIA (n = 17) and symptoms of arthralgia (n = 19) aged 6 to 16 years (56%) followed up at a rheumatology clinic at a tertiary care children's hospital. The most popular types of interventions were prayer, massage therapy, and meditation/ relaxation. In 2007, Rouster-Stevens and colleagues[13] surveyed 52 parents of children with JIA at a pediatric rheumatology clinic that cared for these children from birth to the age of 21 years. CAM was used in the previous 30 days in 92% of the families, including massage therapy, vitamins and other supplements, diets, and stress management techniques. Finally, Feldman and colleagues[11] conducted a preliminary analysis of a cross-sectional study on 118 children with JIA aged 2 to 18 years, followed up at 2 outpatient rheumatology clinics. The study was continued for a 1-year period from 2003 to 2004.[14] In this study, 34% of the patients used CAM, with the most commonly used modalities being naturopathy, acupuncture, chiropractic, and diets. In the longitudinal continuation of this study (n = 182 children with JIA at baseline), 40% of the participants used more than one type of CAM, particularly diets and supplements, chiropractic, and naturopathy. Differences in use of CAM may be explained by questionnaires, each assessing a different range of CAM types because of different definitions of CAM, different time frames, as well as populations with different sociodemographic and disease-related characteristics.

Factors Related to CAM Use

Some parents of children with JIA may seek CAM if they fear side effects of conventional medications and perceive that the child's condition is not improving with such therapy.[14,20] Most parents use CAM to relieve pain in their children.[11,12,20] CAM was also used to improve overall well-being in 20% of the cases.[12]

Factors associated with CAM use in children with JIA include longer disease duration,[10] presence of more than one illness,[10] previous CAM use by parents themselves,[11,14] and parents' perception that medications are not helping.[14] Older age may be associated with CAM use but could also be a reflection of disease duration.[9] In addition, parents who considered themselves as Canadian as opposed to belonging to a specific ethnic group were higher users of CAM according to Feldman's cross-sectional study[11] but not according to the longitudinal analysis of the same cohort by Toupin April and colleagues.[14] Factors associated with the continued use of CAM (use in more than a single 3-month interval) in this population were previous parental use and parents' perceived unhelpfulness of the prescribed medications. Use of CAM also seems to be related to improved psychological functioning in children with arthralgia.[12] Also, according to the 1-year longitudinal study, children who used CAM did not seem to show improved outcomes, at least over this relatively short term but seemed to be more adherent to conventional treatment according to the rheumatologist.[19] Finally, the level of acculturation (ie, language, ethnic identity, cultural heritage, and ethnic interaction) was not found to be associated with CAM use.[12] None of the studies in pediatric rheumatology have examined whether ethnicity was related to the type of CAM used. However, prayer seemed to be used more extensively in a study of Latin American children, whereas vitamins, supplements, and special diets were most commonly used in studies including children from other ethnic backgrounds.

Costs Associated with CAM

None of the studies on JIA mention the financial costs of using CAM. However, one study conducted in Quebec, Canada mentioned the methods of payment for the use of CAM. Among the episodes of CAM use, 69% were paid by parents, 18% were paid by private insurance, 8% were free, 5% were paid by another source, and less than 1% was paid by the provincial universal insurance plan. The CAM treatments that were paid for most often by parents were dietary treatments (90%), chiropractic (81%), and homeopathy (75%), whereas those paid for most often by private insurance were acupuncture (46%), massage (29%), and osteopathy (27%). However, these results depend strongly on the extent of insurance coverage available to each participant, whether public or private. In the general American pediatric population, the average annual amounts spent per person on CAM visits and remedies were $73.40 and $13.06, respectively.[5] Estimates of the 1996 national pediatric population on annual expenditures on CAM visits and remedies were $127 million and $22 million, respectively,[5] with higher costs for children with a chronic condition.

Perceived Effectiveness and Side Effects of CAM

Many parents reported positive results of CAM. Among parents of Latin American children with JIA or arthralgia, 80% thought that CAM was somewhat helpful.[12] Another study[13] showed that the therapies perceived to be the most effective (rated on a 4-point scale from not helpful to very helpful) were support groups, spiritual healing, rubbing menthol-based balm on the joints, and vitamin D. Overall, CAM therapies showed a perception of helpfulness similar to conventional medication but with fewer perceived side effects. Finally, in another study,[14] parents of children with JIA reported that 28% of episodes of use were not beneficial and 23% were somewhat beneficial, while 49% were moderately to highly beneficial, with most CAM types leading to a slight to moderate improvement.

EFFICACY AND SAFETY

According to a systematic search (in the Allied and Complementary Medicine Database [AMED], Cochrane Central Register of Controlled Trials [CENTRAL], EMBASE, MEDLINE) from the earliest date of existence of each database until April 2010 for randomized controlled trials (RCTs) and systematic reviews on the efficacy and safety of CAM in pediatric rheumatology, there seems to be a lack of research. Thus, one is compelled to rely mostly on the few studies conducted in pediatrics and even on the adult literature. Because these studies vary depending on the type of CAM, the 5 domains defined by NCCAM are used to present the extent of the evidence found.[18]

Alternative Medical Systems

Acupuncture

The use of acupuncture is more complicated in children than in adults because of issues such as fear of needles and shortened time of needle insertion due to discomfort.[21] In these cases, acupressure (pressure stimulation at acupuncture locations) seems to be well accepted by younger children. A review of acupuncture efficacy and safety in pediatric patients found some evidence for efficacy and low risk of serious adverse events.[21] However, pediatric data for musculoskeletal pain remained inconclusive because of the poor quality of trials. The incidence of side effects was estimated to be 1.55/100 treatments, with the most commonly reported side effect being puncture redness.[21] The risk of serious adverse events was estimated between 0.05 and 5.36/10000 pediatric treatments.[21] Thus, acupuncture seems to be well tolerated in children in that the incidence of side effects is low and mostly inconsequential. Auricular electroacupuncture has also been studied in adults with rheumatoid arthritis. The 6-week treatment resulted in significant improvements in pain intensity, use of pain medication, the pain disability index, the clinical global impression, and proinflammatory cytokine levels, which were assessed during the study period and 3 months after the end of treatment.[22] Methodological issues exist with many acupuncture studies, especially in pediatrics, including randomization method flaws, small sample sizes, short study duration, and inappropriate selection of outcome measures.[23]

Mind-Body Interventions

Two studies assessed the effect of mind-body interventions, including various relaxation techniques, guided imagery, and meditative breathing, in 21 patients with JIA. Improvements were noted in self-reported pain intensity, whereas no negative treatment effects were reported, but a low adherence to the intervention was found.[24,25] A few studies have also examined biofeedback and hypnosis[26,27] in adult rheumatology, suggesting positive results in measures of pain and sleep outcomes.[26] However, the small sample size and design of these studies preclude any definitive conclusions on the efficacy and safety of these modalities.

Biologically Based Therapies

NHPs

One of the biggest challenges in providing good advice about the use of NHPs is the lack of quality evidence about their safety and efficacy in children. In most cases, few clinical trials have been conducted and little information is available about dosing.

NHP regulations vary tremendously depending on the jurisdiction. In the United States, the Dietary Supplement Health and Education Act of 1994 governs the regulations of NHPs. In general, manufacturers neither need to register their products with the Food and Drug Administration (FDA) nor get an FDA approval before producing or selling dietary supplements.[28] In some cases, adverse events have been associated with NHPs contaminated with pesticides, heavy metals, and toxins. In Canada, the federal department Health Canada implemented regulations to increase the quality assurance of these products. NHPs are, as of 2004, federally regulated as a subcategory of drugs. These NHPs include vitamins, minerals, traditional Chinese medicines, ayurvedic medicines, native North American medicines, traditional herbal remedies, and homeopathic medicines.[29] In Canada, premarket approval in the form of a product license is required for every NHP new to the Canadian market after January 2004. A product license is granted after a review of basic evidence on the efficacy and safety of the product in question. Moreover, there are requirements for manufacturing, packaging, labeling, storing, importing, and distributing.[30] In Germany, all medicines must be approved for sale and are dispensed through a pharmacy. Medicines include chemicals, plants and their parts, animal parts, and microorganisms.[31]

Nutritional supplements Nutritional management of rheumatic diseases is also an important consideration. Nutrient supplementation with products such as fatty acids, antioxidants, zinc, iron, and folate has been studied. Although research supports the use of a balanced diet rich in long-chain n-3 polyunsaturated fatty acids and antioxidants for the management of inflammatory symptoms in rheumatoid arthritis,[32] more research is needed on the benefits of specific nutritional supplementation.[33] Research has been done in children with JIA on the effect of daily calcium (1000 mg) supplementation, suggesting its relevance in the maintenance of physiologic needs and bone mineral density (BMD).[34,35] Calcium supplementation resulted in a small, but statistically significant, increase in total body BMD compared with placebo in children with JIA, and levels of markers of bone physiology were significantly decreased in children with JIA receiving calcium supplementation.[34,35]

Herbal medicine When evaluating the extent of the research in herbal medicines, it is important to note that herbal products are often combination formulations with many ingredients, which may differ in their active ingredients and standardization. RCTs of herbal interventions must adequately describe details of the herbal products used.[36] In fact, the efficacy and safety of herbal products vary according to several factors, such as the geographic source of the plant material, climate in which they were grown, time of harvest, as well as part of the plant used and the choice of extraction method.[37] It is often difficult to pool data from RCTs into a systematic review, especially in the case of herbal therapies, because of variations in these key parameters. There is also the possibility of interactions between herbal products and drugs (eg, the possible diminished efficacy of corticosteroids and methotrexate because of the use of products from Echinacea)[38] and undesirable effects (such as bleeding and interaction with anesthesia) of certain herbal products (eg, St John's wort, garlic, and Ginkgo biloba) during surgery.[39]

Some herbal medicines have shown promise for reducing pain and inflammation in rheumatic diseases in adults. There is some encouraging research on compounds such as γ-linolenic acid plants such as Harpagophytum procumbens (devil's claw), Tanacetum parthenium (feverfew), Uncaria tomentosa (cat's claw), Urtica diocia (stinging nettles) and Zingiber officinale (ginger).[40,41] However, more high-quality research is needed, especially to examine the effects in children. The most commonly studied herb for rheumatoid arthritis is Tripterygium wilfordii (TWF), sometimes called the thunder god vine.[40] In adults, studies have shown clinical improvements in the number of tender joints and swollen joints, morning stiffness, physical global assessment, as well as a change in erythrocyte sedimentation rate and C-reactive protein.[40] A study was conducted with TWF on 59 patients with rheumatic diseases, 6 of whom were classified as originally having JIA. All patients with JIA reported decreased pain and swelling as well as improved range of motion.[42]

Manipulative and Body-Based Methods

Manual therapy

Spinal manipulation, most often performed by chiropractors, is a manual therapy applied to body tissues with a therapeutic intent to treat neuromuscular problems that stem from a mechanical disability. Although chiropractic care is common among children, efficacy and safety data are scarce.[43,44] There is a lack of RCTs in children with musculoskeletal conditions. Also, case studies report complications (such as pain, loss of consciousness, and delayed treatment of another disease) from spinal manipulation, but the true adverse event incidence is unknown. Methodological issues relate to poor evaluation of adverse events in randomized trials, lack of sufficient pediatric training for some therapists, and predisposing complications.[43]

Massage therapy

Massage combines tactile and kinesthetic stimulation of the body performed in sequential application. Evidence suggests promise for the use of massage therapy for reducing pain in JIA. Children with mild to moderate JIA who were massaged by their parents showed immediate decreases in anxiety and cortisol levels. After 1 month, the children's incidence and severity of pain decreased, measured by the physician's assessment and the parent's and child's assessments as per the Varni/Thompson Pediatric Pain Questionaire.[45] Also, adverse events may be a concern but are extremely rare when massage is provided by a trained massage therapist.[46] Although results are promising, further research is needed on the long-term effects and underlying mechanisms.

REFLECTION ON THE STATE OF RESEARCH

Despite the common use of CAM in pediatric rheumatology (34%–92%) and its perceived effectiveness, there is still uncertainty as to its efficacy and safety. Results seem promising for some treatments such as massage, mind-body interventions (eg, guided imagery and meditative breathing) and some NHPs (eg, calcium supplements and TWF). However, there is a paucity of good-quality evidence for most therapies and products intended for use in pediatric rheumatology. In order to move forward, some methodological issues in current research need to be highlighted.

First, there is no consensus regarding the definition of CAM. Efforts are being made to determine which terms are the most adequate and which definition of CAM should be agreed upon.[47] Initial findings of a systematic review also suggest that there is no well-validated questionnaire that adequately assesses CAM use in pediatric patients,[48] making it difficult to compare the results of different studies. Thus, efforts should be made to develop and validate instruments assessing the use of CAM as well as other important aspects of CAM relevant to pediatric clinical and research settings. Because children are the ones who must adhere to a panoply of treatments, it may be important for these instruments to evaluate how they are involved in the decision-making process to use CAM as well as the effect of these treatments on their and their family's lives. Such instruments would ensure that results from different studies could be compared. Furthermore, an instrument that could be used in clinical practice may help assess CAM use in a more systematic way, thus improving communication between families and their health care providers. Other tools that could be used to improve knowledge transfer and improve patients' self-management include decision aids and self-management programs.

Qualitative methods and mixed methods (both qualitative and quantitative methods) are also lacking and may be useful in order to get a full understanding of how parents and children cope with a chronic disease and follow their medical regimen. It may be especially important to describe patterns of longitudinal CAM use, given the chronic aspect of JIA, the variability of the disease over time, and the fact that using CAM could interfere with the standard treatments. These studies may help in identifying the approach to use with patients and their families in order to improve the outcomes of both conventional care and CAM.

Finally, in pediatric rheumatology, there is a lack of high-quality RCTs as well as studies about the mechanisms of action of CAM, especially in the field of NHPs. Studies could help determine the manner in which CAM should be administered (frequency, duration, dosage, and timing of intervention compared with conventional care) in order to promote the most relevant outcomes according to patients. This information would lead to the conduct of well-designed RCTs, which would in turn shed light on their efficacy and safety. Economic evaluations of the use of these treatments should also be performed in a more systematic way in order to evaluate their cost-effectiveness.

AVENUES FOR CLINICAL PRACTICE

The scientific literature underscores the importance for health care providers to be aware of their patients' use of CAM and to be knowledgeable about potential benefits and harms. Before making a judgment about the CAM modalities, health care providers should have access to the best-updated scientific evidence and, in the presence of a paucity of data as exists in pediatric rheumatology, they should keep an open dialogue with their patients concerning these treatments in order to monitor their use.

ACKNOWLEDGMENTS

The authors would like to thank Ms Tamara Rader, MLIS for designing and conducting the literature search, Dr Sunita Vohra, Erin Ueffing, and Ian Disend for reviewing the article.

REFERENCES

1. Kemper KJ, O'Connor KG. Pediatricians' recommendations for complementary and alternative medical (CAM) therapies. Ambul Pediatr 2004;4:482–7.
2. Kemper KJ, Vohra S, Walls R. American Academy of Pediatrics. The use of complementary and alternative medicine in pediatrics. Pediatrics 2008;122: 1374–86.
3. Spigelblatt L, Laine-Ammara G, Pless IB, et al. The use of alternative medicine by children. Pediatrics 1994;94:811–4.
4. Simpson N, Roman K. Complementary medicine use in children: extent and reasons. A population-based study. Br J Gen Pract 2001;51(472):914–6.
5. Yussman SM, Ryan SA, Auinger P, et al. Visits to complementary and alternative medicine providers by children and adolescents in the United States. Ambul Pediatr 2004;4:429–35.
6. Maclennan AH, Myers SP, Taylor AW. The continuing use of complementary and alternative medicine in South Australia: costs and beliefs in 2004. Med J Aust 2006;184(1):27–31.
7. Post-White J, Fitzgerald M, Hageness S, et al. Complementary and alternative medicine use in children with cancer and general and specialty pediatrics. J Pediatr Oncol Nurs 2009;26(1):7–15.
8. Wilson K. Use of complementary medicine and dietary supplements among U.S. adolescents. J Adolesc Health 2006;38:385–94.
9. Southwood TR, Malleson PN, Roberts-Thomson PJ, et al. Unconventional remedies used for patients with juvenile arthritis. Pediatrics 1990;85:150–4.
10. Hagen LE, Schneider R, Stephens D, et al. Use of complementary and alternative medicine by pediatric rheumatology patients. Arthritis Rheum 2003;49:3–6.
11. Feldman DE, Duffy C, De Civita M, et al. Factors associated with the use of complementary and alternative medicine in juvenile idiopathic arthritis. Arthritis Rheum 2004;51:527–32.

12. Zebracki K, Holzman K, Bitter KJ, et al. Brief report: use of complementary and alternative medicine and psychological functioning in Latino children with juvenile idiopathic arthritis or arthralgia. J Pediatr Psychol 2007;32:1006–10.
13. Rouster-Stevens K, Nageswaran S, Arcury TA, et al. How do parents of children with juvenile idiopathic arthritis (JIA) perceive their therapies? BMC Complement Altern Med 2008;8:25.
14. Toupin April K, Ehrmann Feldman D, Zunzunegui MV, et al. Longitudinal analysis of complementary and alternative health care use in children with juvenile idiopathic arthritis. Complement Ther Med 2009;17:208–15.
15. Cockayne NL, Duguid M, Shenfield GM. Health professionals rarely record history of complementary and alternative medicines. Br J Clin Pharmacol 2005;59:254–8.
16. Kroll T, Barlow JH, Shaw K. Treatment adherence in juvenile rheumatoid arthritis– a review. Scand J Rheumatol 1999;28:10–8.
17. Fearon J. A reflective overview of complementary therapies for children 1995–2005. Complement Ther Clin Pract 2005;11:32–6.
18. National Center for Complementary and Alternative Medicine Web site. 2004. Available at: www.nccam.nih.gov/health/whatiscam. Accessed May 31, 2010.
19. Toupin-April K, Feldman DE, Zunzunegui MV, et al. Is complementary and alternative healthcare use associated with better outcomes in children with juvenile idiopathic arthritis? J Rheumatol 2009;36:2302–7.
20. Toupin April K, Ehrmann Feldman D, Zunzunegui MV. Why do children with juvenile idiopathic arthritis (JIA) use complementary and alternative health care (CAHC)? J Complement Integr Med 2006;3:36.
21. Jindal V, Ge A, Mansky PJ. Safety and efficacy of acupuncture in children: a review of the evidence. J Pediatr Hematol Oncol 2008;30:431–42.
22. Bernateck M, Becker M, Schwake C, et al. Adjuvant auricular electroacupuncture and autogenic training in rheumatoid arthritis: a randomized controlled trial. Auricular acupuncture and autogenic training in rheumatoid arthritis. Forsch Komplementmed 2008;15:187–93.
23. Casimiro L, Barnsley L, Brosseau L, et al. Acupuncture and electroacupuncture for the treatment of rheumatoid arthritis. Cochrane Database Syst Rev 2005;4: CD003788.
24. Lavigne JV, Ross CK, Berry SL, et al. Evaluation of a psychological treatment package for treating pain in juvenile rheumatoid arthritis. Arthritis Care Res 1992;5:101–10.
25. Walco GA, Varni JW, Ilowite NT. Cognitive-behavioral pain management in children with juvenile rheumatoid arthritis. Pediatrics 1992;89:1075–9.
26. Achterberg J, McGraw P, Lawlis. Rheumatoid arthritis: a study of relaxation and temperature biofeedback training as an adjunctive therapy. Biofeedback Self Regul 1981;6(2):207–23.
27. Horton JR. Clinical hypnosis in the treatment of rheumatoid arthritis. Psychologische Beitrage 1994;36:205–12.
28. Dietary Supplements: FDA U.S. Food and Drug Administration. 2010.
29. Government of Canada. Natural Health Product Regulations. Food and Drugs Act. 2010.
30. Health Canada. About Natural Health Product Regulation in Canada. 3-4-2009.
31. Harrison JR. International regulation of natural health products. Boca Raton (FL): Universal Publishers; 2008.
32. Goldberg RJ, Katz J. Meta-analysis of the analgesic effects of omega-3 polyunsaturated fatty acid supplementation for inflammatory joint pain. Pain 2007; 129(1–2):210–23.

33. Rennie KL, Rennie KL. Nutritional management of rheumatoid arthritis: a review of the evidence. J Hum Nutr Diet 2003;16(2):97–109.

34. Carrasco R, Lovell DJ, Giannini EH, et al. Biochemical markers of bone turnover associated with calcium supplementation in children with juvenile rheumatoid arthritis: results of a double-blind, placebo-controlled intervention trial. Arthritis Rheum 2008;58:3932–40.

35. Lovell DJ, Glass D, Ranz J, et al. A randomized controlled trial of calcium supplementation to increase bone mineral density in children with juvenile rheumatoid arthritis. Arthritis Rheum 2006;54:2235–42.

36. Moher D, Soeken K, Sampson M, et al. Assessing the quality of reports of systematic reviews in pediatric complementary and alternative medicine. BMC Pediatr 2002;2:3.

37. Wolsko PM, Solondz DK, Phillips RS, et al. Lack of herbal supplement characterization in published randomized controlled trials. Am J Med 2005;118:1087–93.

38. Miller LG. Herbal medicinals: selected clinical considerations focusing on known or potential drug-herb interactions. Arch Intern Med 1998;158:2200–11.

39. Crowe S, Lyons B. Herbal medicine use by children presenting for ambulatory anesthesia and surgery. Paediatr Anaesth 2004;14:916–9.

40. Setty AR, Sigal LH. Herbal medications commonly used in the practice of rheumatology: mechanisms of action, efficacy, and side effects. Semin Arthritis Rheum 2005;34:773–84.

41. Soeken KLE, Soeken KL. Selected CAM therapies for arthritis-related pain: the evidence from systematic reviews. Clin J Pain 2004;20(1):13–8.

42. Ju-Ling G, Zhi-guo G, An-chang Z, et al. Radix Tripterygium wilfordii Hook f in rheumatoid arthritis, ankylosing spondylitis and juvenile rheumatoid arthritis. Chin Med J 1986;99(4):317–20.

43. Vohra S, Johnston BC, Cramer K, et al. Adverse events associated with pediatric spinal manipulation: a systematic review [structured abstract]. Pediatrics 2007; 119:e275–83.

44. Hestbaek L, Stochkendahl MJ. The evidence base for chiropractic treatment of musculoskeletal conditions in children and adolescents: the emperor's new suit? Chiropr Osteopat 2010;18:15.

45. Field T, Hernandez-Reif M, Seligman S, et al. Juvenile rheumatoid arthritis: benefits from massage therapy. J Pediatr Psychol 1997;22:607–17.

46. Beider S, Mahrer NE, Gold JI. Pediatric massage therapy: an overview for clinicians. Pediatr Clin North Am 2007;54:1025–41.

47. Gaboury I, Toupin April K, Verhoef M. Is the label CAM still adequate? A Delphi survey. In: Proceedings of the Fifth International Congress on Complementary Medicine Research. Tromso (Norway), May 19, 2010.

48. Toupin April K, Byrne A, Dhaliwal B, et al. A systematic review of complementary and alternative health care measures in pediatrics: are measures asking the right questions in the right way? In: Proceedings of the Fifth International Congress on Complementary Medicine Research. Tromso (Norway), May 19, 2010.

Herbal Medicine in the Treatment of Rheumatic Diseases

Edzard Ernst, MD, PhD, FMedSci, FSB, FRCP, FRCPEd

KEYWORDS

• Herbal medicine • Rheumatic disease • Antiinflammatory
• Osteoarthritis

Herbal medicines are popular, self-prescribed treatments for rheumatic conditions. A recent US survey suggested that approximately 90% of arthritic patients use alternative therapies such as herbal medicines.[1] Many patients try multiple alternative treatments.[2] The reasons for this high level of popularity are complex[1] and include the following factors:

- Conventional medicine is not always optimally effective.
- Drugs frequently have adverse effects.
- Herbal medicines are heavily promoted, for example, by the popular press, Internet sites, popular books, and celebrities.
- Herbal medicines are widely available, usually marketed as food supplements.
- Exaggerated claims are often made regarding their efficacy.
- The public tends to view herbs as natural and thus devoid of risks.
- Most consumers can afford the extra costs for herbal medicines.

As more patients start using alternative medicine, conventional health care practitioners increasingly feel the need to acquaint themselves with herbal medicines.[3,4] This article provides a brief overview of the evidence on herbal medicines for 4 common rheumatic conditions: back pain, fibromyalgia, osteoarthritis, and rheumatoid arthritis. Nonherbal supplements, for example, vitamins or glucosamine, were excluded. This overview is based mainly on the author's systematic assessments of these conditions,[5–7] supplemented with relevant, more recent data.

BACK PAIN

Several herbal medicines are supported by promising results in terms of alleviating musculoskeletal pain, and many patients who also use such treatments perceive

Complementary Medicine, Peninsula Medical School, University of Exeter, 25 Victoria Park Road, Exeter, EX2 4NT, UK
E-mail address: Edzard.Ernst@pms.ac.uk

Rheum Dis Clin N Am 37 (2011) 95–102
doi:10.1016/j.rdc.2010.11.004
0889-857X/11/$ – see front matter © 2011 Elsevier Inc. All rights reserved.

them to be effective.[8] The remedy that has been most thoroughly investigated, specifically for back pain, is devil's claw (*Harpagophytum procumbens*), which has antiinflammatory and analgesic actions. A systematic review included 4 randomized clinical trials (RCTs) of devil's claw for back pain.[9] The methodological quality of these studies was mostly good, and collectively their results were encouraging. The review concluded that devil's claw, at a dose of 100 mg hapagside per day, is an effective symptomatic treatment of back pain (**Table 1**).[9]

Other herbal medicines that have shown promise in recent clinical trials include willow bark (*Salix alba*) extracts and capsicum creams (see **Table 1**).[10] Willow bark contains salicin (aspirin was derived from willow bark), which has analgesic and antipyretic effects. Capsicum is a powerful skin irritant and acts as a counterirritant relieving pain.

FIBROMYALGIA

The UK Arthritis Research Campaign (ARC) recently initiated a systematic review of herbal medicines as a treatment of fibromyalgia.[7] Seven clinical trials were located. The effects of oral anthocyanidins and topical capsaicin demonstrated an improvement in sleep disturbance and tenderness, respectively, but not in other end points such as pain. For orally administered soy, the evidence was negative, but only 1 study was found. The ARC review[7] concluded that "there is insufficient evidence" for any herbal medicine as a treatment of fibromyalgia. For the plethora of Chinese herbal medicines, the evidence is, generally speaking, of poor methodological quality and therefore inconclusive.[11,12] In particular, many studies are underpowered, poorly controlled, and poorly reported.

OSTEOARTHRITIS

A Cochrane review assessed all placebo-controlled RCTs of herbal analgesic treatments of osteoarthritis pain (see **Table 1**).[13] A total of 5 trials using 4 different herbal medicines were identified. The data from the 2 studies that tested avocado-soybean unsaponifiables (ASUs) were pooled, which provided some encouraging evidence. ASUs inhibit interleukin-1 synthesis and have antiinflammatory effects.[5] Another systematic review identified 4 double-blind, placebo-controlled RCTs of ASUs.[14] It concluded that, mainly because of the paucity of the rigorous clinical trials, the clinical evidence is, at present, not fully convincing (see **Table 1**).

A systematic review assessed the effects of devil's claw for osteoarthritic pain.[9] It included RCTs, quasi-RCTs, and non-RCTs and concluded that there was limited evidence to support the use of an ethanolic extract containing harpagoside, 30 mg/d, in the treatment of knee and hip osteoarthritis. There was a moderate evidence of effectiveness for the use of a devil's claw powder containing 60 mg harpagoside in the treatment of osteoarthritis of the knee, hip, and spine (see **Table 1**).

A systematic review assessed all RCTs of ginger (*Zingiber officinalis*).[15] Ginger contains a wide range of pharmacologically active ingredients that have been shown to exhibit antiinflammatory activity. Only 1 small RCT (*n* = 56) was identified in the review. It reported no difference compared with placebo for Lequesne index and pain caused by osteoarthritis of the knee. However, a more recent, large (*n* = 247), double-blind RCT found a reduction in pain.[16] Another double-blind RCT reported superiority of ginger over placebo in terms of pain relief at the end of 6 months.[17] Another RCT reported superiority of ginger extract over placebo but no difference between ginger and ibuprofen in the short term.[18]

Table 1
Systematic reviews of herbal medicine

Type of Herbal Medication	Condition	Number and Average Methodological Quality of Primary Studies	Conclusion	References
Devil's claw (*Harpagophytum procumens*)	Back pain, OA	4 Good	This remedy is an effective symptomatic treatment of low back pain and OA	9
Any	Back pain	10 Good	Good evidence exists for several herbal medicines	10
Any Chinese herbal medicine	Fibromyalgia	25 Poor	Studies are of insufficient methodology rigor	11
Any*	OA	5 Satisfactory	Current evidence is insufficient for a reliable assessment of efficacy	13
ASU	OA	4 Good	ASU is effective for the symptomatic treatment of OA	14
Any	OA	25 Mixed	Some encouraging evidence	15
Phytodolor	Arthritis pain	6 Good	Positive evidence from several rigorous studies	19
Rose hip (*Rosa canina*)	OA	4 Mixed	Evidence is positive but not strong	20
Ayurvedic herbal medicines	RhA	7 Moderate	The existing data are unconvincing	34
Any	RhA	20 Good	Positive evidence only for γ-linoleic acid	38
Thunder god vine (*Tripterygium wilfordii*)	RhA	2 Good	Evidence for efficacy is encouraging, but there are important adverse effects	41

Abbreviations: ASU, avocado-soybean unsaponifiables; OA, osteoarthritis; RhA, rheumatoid arthritis.
* Cochrane review.

The efficacy of Phytodolor (a proprietary preparation which contains *Populus tremula*, *Fraxinus excelsior*, and *Solidago virgaurea*) in painful arthritic conditions has been assessed in several studies. Several of the constituents are known to have antiinflammatory effects. A systematic review identified 6 double-blind RCTs (see **Table 1**).[19] These trials suggest pain reduction, increase in mobility, and a reduction in the consumption of nonsteroidal antiinflammatory drugs.

A systematic review of rose hip (*Rosa canina*) preparations identified 4 relevant RCTs. The mode of action is not entirely clear, but antiinflammatory effects are likely to play a role. The review concluded that moderate evidence exists for the use of a powder of the seeds and husks of a rose hip subspecies in patients with osteoarthritis of the hip and knee.[20]

SKI 306X is a purified extract from a mixture of 3 herbs (*Clematis mandshurica*, *Trichosanthes kirilowii*, and *Prunella vulgaris*). The mechanisms of action are uncertain; most likely they involve antiinflammatory effects. The extract was tested in patients with osteoarthritis of the knee and was found to be superior to placebo when pain was measured with the visual analog scale and Lequesne index.[21] In a trial that compared the herbal mixture with diclofenac, 300 mg/d, both preparations showed similar effects on pain.[22]

Single RCTs, which require independent replications, exist for willow bark (*Salix* spp),[23] the herbal mixtures Reumalex[24] and Tipi,[25] a herbomineral formulation,[26] Gitadyl,[27] Eazimov,[28] stinging nettle (*Urtica dioica*),[29] boswellia (*Boswellia serrata*),[30] and the Chinese mixed preparations Duhuo Jisheng Wan,[31] Qianggu,[32] and Garcinia kola.[33] The mechanisms of action involved are diverse but typically involve antiinflammatory effects of the herbal ingredients.

RHEUMATOID ARTHRITIS

A systematic review assessed the evidence from all RCTs testing the effectiveness of ayurvedic medicine (see **Table 1**).[34] In general, the quality of the primary studies was disappointing. Many studies were poorly reported and associated with small sample sizes and high risks of bias. There was a paucity of RCTs of ayurvedic medicines for rheumatoid arthritis and a near total lack of independent replications. Therefore, it would be unwise to recommend such treatments to patients suffering from rheumatoid arthritis.

A double-blind RCT assessed the short-term effects of a cannabis-based medicine (Sativex) in 58 patients.[35] Cannabis has well-documented analgesic effects. In comparison with placebo, cannabis produced improvements in pain on movement, pain at rest, and quality of sleep.

An extract of cat's claw (*Uncaria tomentosa*) was tested in 40 patients treated with sulfasalazine or hydroxychloroquine.[36] Twenty-four weeks of treatment with the extract resulted in a modest reduction in the number of painful joints compared with placebo. This study was small and preliminary; the results require independent replication.

A Cochrane review of herbal treatments for rheumatoid arthritis concluded that there seems to be beneficial effects on pain from γ-linoleic acid, although further studies are required to establish optimal dosage and duration of treatment.[37] A more recent assessment of the evidence includes more trial data and largely corroborates these findings, moderately supporting the use of γ-linoleic acid for reducing pain, tender joint count, and stiffness (see **Table 1**).[38] The antiinflammatory effects of γ-linoleic acid are well documented.

Several herbal mixtures have been tested in clinical trials, with positive results for patients with rheumatoid arthritis. Of these preparations, only Phytodolor has been subjected to independently replicated clinical trials.[19] Collectively, these data from the pre–tumor necrosis factor era suggest that this herbal mixture is effective in alleviating pain of rheumatoid arthritis.

Thunder god vine (*Tripterygium wilfordii*) is often recommended in traditional Chinese medicine for a large range of conditions. RCTs suggested antiinflammatory properties and effects in reducing the objective signs and subjective symptoms of rheumatoid arthritis.[39,40] A systematic review assessed the totality of the available evidence and concluded that, because of the limited number of available RCTs and the reported serious adverse effects, this medicine cannot be recommended for use.[41]

Other single RCTs report some positive results for rose hip,[42] pine bark extract,[43] biqi,[44] garlic (*Allium sativum*),[45] tong luo kai bi tablets,[46] and various Chinese mixtures.[22,47,48] The mechanisms of actions of these preparations are diverse, but usually, antiinflammatory actions are thought to cause the clinical effects. The results require independent replications. Conflicting results exist for Indian frankincense (*Boswellia serrata*)[37,49] and willow bark extract.[23,50]

COMMENT

This brief overview suggests that some encouraging evidence exists for some herbal medicines as treatments of the 4 common rheumatic conditions mentioned earlier. It also highlights the relative paucity and often disappointing methodological quality of the primary studies. Further caveats should be mentioned; they include the following points:

- Some herbal medicines are associated with serious adverse effects.[51]
- Herbal medicines are not always of adequate quality; particular problems are contamination and adulteration.[52,53]
- Interactions with prescribed drugs may cause problems.[54]
- Most herbalists practice individualized herbalism, yet for this approach, there is no good evidence of effectiveness.[55]

The field of herbal medicine is thus fraught with uncertainty. Vis à vis patients' seemingly insatiable appetite for such remedies, it would seem wise to conduct more and better research into this area, so that one can tell with reasonable certainty which herbal treatments generate more good than harm for which patient groups.

REFERENCES

1. Herman CJ, Allen P, Hunt WC, et al. Use of complementary therapies among primary care clinic patients with arthritis. Prev Chronic Dis 2004;1(4):A12.
2. Efthimiou P, Kukar M, Mackenzie CR. Complementary and alternative medicine in rheumatoid arthritis: no longer the last resort! HSS J 2009. [Epub ahead of print].
3. Manek NJ, Crowson CS, Ottenberg AL, et al. What rheumatologists in the United States think of complementary and alternative medicine: results of a national survey. BMC Complement Altern Med 2010;10:5.
4. Osborn C, Baxter GD, Barlas P, et al. Complementary and alternative medicine and rheumatology nurses: a survey of current use and perceptions. Nurs Times 2004;9(2):110–9.
5. Ernst E, Pittler MH, Wider B, et al. The desktop guide to complementary and alternative medicine. 2nd edition. Edinburgh (UK): Elsevier Mosby; 2006.
6. Ernst E, Pittler MH, Wider B, et al. Complementary therapies for pain management. An evidence-based approach. London: Elsevier; 2007.

7. De Silva V, El-Metwally A, Ernst E, et al. Evidence for the efficacy of complementary and alternative medicine in the management of fibromyalgia: a systematic review. Rheumatology (Oxford) 2010;49(6):1063–8.

8. Kanodia AK, Legedza AT, Davis RB, et al. Perceived benefit of complementary and alternative medicine (CAM) for back pain: a national survey. J Am Board Fam Med 2010;23(3):354–62.

9. Gagnier JJ, Chrubasik S, Manheimer E. *Harpagophytum procumbens* for osteoarthritis and low back pain: a systematic review. BMC Complement Altern Med 2004;4:13.

10. Gagnier JJ, van Tulder MW, Berman B, et al. Herbal medicine for low back pain: a Cochrane review. Spine 2007;32(1):82–92.

11. Zheng L, Faber K. Review of the Chinese medical approach to the management of fibromyalgia. Curr Pain Headache Rep 2005;9(5):307–12.

12. Cao H, Liu J, Lewith GT. Traditional Chinese medicine for treatment of fibromyalgia: a systematic review of randomized controlled trials. J Altern Complement Med 2010;16(4):397–409.

13. Little CV, Parsons T, Logan S. Herbal therapy for treating osteoarthritis. Cochrane Database Syst Rev 2000;4:CD002947.

14. Ernst E. Avocado-soybean unsaponifiables (ASU) for osteoarthritis – a systematic review. Clin Rheumatol 2003;22:285–8.

15. Long L, Ernst E, Soeken K. Herbal medicines for the treatment of osteoarthritis: a systematic review. Rheumatology(Oxford) 2001;40:779–93.

16. Altman RD, Marcussen KC. Effects of a ginger extract on knee pain in patients with osteoarthritis. Arthritis Rheum 2001;44:2531–8.

17. Wigler I, Grotto I, Caspi D, et al. The effects of Zintona EC (a ginger extract) on symptomatic gonarthritis. Osteoarthr Cartil 2003;11:783–9.

18. Haghighi M, Khalvat A, Toliat T, et al. Comparing the effects of ginger (*Zingiber officinale*) extract and ibuprofen on patients with osteoarthritis. Arch Iran Med 2005;8:267–71.

19. Ernst E. The efficacy of Phytodolor for the treatment of musculoskeletal pain – a systematic review of randomized clinical trials. Nat Med J 1999;2:14–7.

20. Chrubasik C, Duke RK, Chrubasik S. The evidence for clinical efficacy of rose hip and seed: a systematic review. Phytother Res 2006;20(1):1–3.

21. Jung YB, Roh KJ, Jung JA, et al. Effect of SKI306X, a new herbal anti-arthritic agent, in patients with osteoarthritis of the knee: a double-blind placebo controlled study. Am J Chin Med 2001;29:485–91.

22. Lung YB, Seong SC, Lee MC, et al. A four-week, randomized, double-blind trial of the efficacy and safety of SKI306X: a herbal anti-arthritic agent versus diclofenac in osteoarthritis of the knee. Am J Chin Med 2004;32(2): 291–301.

23. Biegert C, Wagner I, Ludtke R, et al. Efficacy and safety of willow bark extract in the treatment of osteoarthritis and rheumatoid arthritis: results of 2 randomized double-blind trials. J Rheumatol 2004;31:2121–30.

24. Mills SY, Jacoby RK, Chacksfield M, et al. Effect of a proprietary herbal medicine on the relief of chronic arthritic pain: a double-blind study. Br J Rheumatol 1996; 35:874–8.

25. Ferraz MB, Pereira RB, Iwata NM, et al. Tipi. A popular analgesic tea: a double-blind cross-over trial in osteoarthritis. Clin Exp Rheumatol 1991;9:205–12.

26. Kulkarni RR, Patki PS, Jog VP, et al. Treatment of osteoarthritis with a herbomineral formulation: a double-blind, placebo-controlled, cross-over study. J Ethnopharmacol 1991;33:91–5.

27. Ryttig K, Schlamowitz PV, Warnoe O, et al. [Gitadyl verus ibuprofen in patients with osteoarthritis. The result of a double-blind, randomized cross-over study]. Ugeskr Laeger 1991;153:2298–9 [in Danish].
28. Biswas NR, Biswas K, Pandey M, et al. Treatment of osteoarthritis, rheumatoid arthritis and non-specific arthritis with a herbal drug: a double-blind, active drug controlled parallel study. JK Pract 1998;5:129–32.
29. Randall C, Randall H, Dobbs F, et al. Randomized controlled trial of nettle sting for treatment of base-of-thumb pain. J R Soc Med 2000;93:305–9.
30. Kimmatkar N, Thawani V, Hingorani L, et al. Efficacy and tolerability of *Boswellia serrata* extract in treatment of osteoarthritis of knee – a randomized double blind placebo controlled trial. Phytomedicine 2003;10:3–7.
31. Teekachunhatean S, Kunanusorn P, Rojanasthien N, et al. Chinese herbal recipe versus diclofenac in symptomatic treatment of osteoarthritis of the knee: a randomized controlled trial [ISRCTN70292892]. BMC Complement Altern Med 2004;4:19.
32. Ruan XY, Liu YL, Peng ZL, et al. Effect of qianggu capsule on the effective range of motion of knee joint in postmenopausal women with knee osteoarthritis. Chin J Clin Rehabil 2005;9:170–1.
33. Adegbehingbe OO, Adesanya SA, Idowu TO, et al. Clinical effects of *Garcinia kola* in knee osteoarthritis. J Orthop Surg Res 2008;3:34.
34. Park J, Ernst E. Ayurvedic medicine for rheumatoid arthritis: a systematic review. Semin Arthritis Rheum 2005;34:705–13.
35. Blake DR, Robson P, Ho M, et al. Preliminary assessment of the efficacy, tolerability and safety of a cannabis-based medicine (Sativex) in the treatment of pain caused by rheumatoid arthritis. Rheumatology (Oxford) 2006;45(1):50–2.
36. Mur E, Hartig F, Eibl G, et al. Randomized double blind trial of an extract from the pentacyclic alkaloid-chemotype of *Uncaria tomentosa* for the treatment of rheumatoid arthritis. J Rheumatol 2002;29:678–81.
37. Little CV, Parsons T, Logan S. Herbal therapy for treating rheumatoid arthritis. Cochrane Database Syst Rev 2000;4:CD002948.
38. Cameron M, Gagnier JJ, Little CV, et al. Evidence of effectiveness of herbal medicinal products in the treatment of arthritis. Part 2: Rheumatoid arthritis. Phytother Res 2009;23(12):1647–62.
39. Cibere J, Deng Z, Lin Y, et al. A randomized double blind, placebo controlled trial of topical *Tripterygium wilfordii* in rheumatoid arthritis: reanalysis using logistic regression. J Rheumatol 2003;30:465–7.
40. Tao X, Younger J, Fan FZ, et al. Benefit of an extract of *Tripterygium wilfordii* Hook F in patients with rheumatoid arthritis: a double-blind, placebo-controlled study. Arthritis Rheum 2002;46:1735–43.
41. Canter PH, Lee HS, Ernst E. A systematic review of randomised clinical trials of *Tripterygium wilfordii* for rheumatoid arthritis. Phytomedicine 2006;13:371–7.
42. Willich SN, Rossnagel K, Roll S, et al. Rose hip herbal remedy in patients with rheumatoid arthritis – a randomised controlled trial. Phytomedicine 2010;17(2):87–93.
43. Cisár P, Jány R, Waczulíková I, et al. Effect of pine bark extract (Pycnogenol) on symptoms of knee osteoarthritis. Phytother Res 2008;22(8):1087–92.
44. Liu W, Zhang L, Xu Z. [Clinical observation on treatment of rheumatoid arthritis with biqi capsule]. Zhongguo Zhong Xi Yi Jie He Za Zhi 2006;26(2):157–9 [in Chinese].
45. Denisov LN, Andrianova IV, Timofeeva SS. [Garlic effectiveness in rheumatoid arthritis]. Ter Arkh 1999;71:55–8 [in Russian].

46. Shi Y, Zhang H, Du X, et al. A double blind observation for therapeutic effects of the tong luo kai bi tablets on rheumatoid arthritis. J Tradit Chin Med 1999;19(3): 166–72.
47. Song YW, Lee EY, Koh EM, et al. Assessment of comparative pain relief and tolerability of SKI306X compared with celecoxib in patients with rheumatoid arthritis: a 6-week, multicenter, randomized, double-blind, double-dummy, phase III, noninferiority clinical trial. Clin Ther 2007;29(5):862–73.
48. Li EK, Tam LS, Wong CK, et al. Safety and efficacy of *Ganoderma lucidum* (lingzhi) and San Miao San supplementation in patients with rheumatoid arthritis: a double-blind, randomized, placebo-controlled pilot trial. Arthritis Rheum 2007;57(7):1143–50.
49. Sengupta K, Alluri KV, Satish AR, et al. A double blind, randomized, placebo controlled study of the efficacy and safety of 5-Loxin for treatment of osteoarthritis of the knee. Arthritis Res Ther 2008;10(4):R85.
50. Beer AM, Wegener T. Willow bark extract (*Salicis cortex*) for gonarthrosis and coxarthrosis – results of a cohort study with a control group. Phytomedicine 2008;15:907–13.
51. Ernst E. Complementary and alternative medicine. In: Dukes MNG, editor. Meyler's side effects of drugs, vols. 2 & 3. Amsterdam: Elsevier; 2006. p. 886–99.
52. Ernst E, Thompson Coon J. Heavy metals in traditional Chinese medicines: a systematic review. Clin Pharmacol Ther 2001;70:497–504.
53. Ernst E. Adulteration of Chinese herbal medicines with synthetic drugs: a systematic review. J Intern Med 2002;252:107–13.
54. Izzo AA, Ernst E. Interactions between herbal medicines and prescribed drugs: an updated systematic review. Drugs 2009;69(13):1777–98.
55. Guo R, Canter PH, Ernst E. A systematic review of randomised clinical trials of individualised herbal medicine in any indication. Postgrad Med J 2007;83:633–7.

Glucosamine and Chondroitin Sulfate

Karla L. Miller, MD[a],*, Daniel O. Clegg, MD[a,b]

KEYWORDS

• Glucosamine • Chondroitin sulfate • Osteoarthritis • Knee

Glucosamine is a hexosamine sugar that is naturally produced in humans. It is an important precursor in the biosynthesis of many connective tissue macromolecules such as hyaluronic acid, proteoglycans, glycosaminoglycans (GAGs), glycolipids, and glycoproteins. Chondroitin sulfate is a prominent GAG found in articular cartilage. Its hydrophilic properties enable the articular cartilage to absorb relatively large quantities of water thereby conveying and absorbing compressive forces on the cartilage. Glucosamine and chondroitin sulfate have gained popularity in recent years as potential therapeutic agents for osteoarthritis (OA), as a major manifestation of this disease is failure of articular hyaline cartilage.[1]

OA is a chronic, progressive, degenerative, articular disease that is particularly common in weight-bearing joints. OA is the most prominent form of arthritis; its prevalence increases dramatically with age.[2] OA can lead to significant pain, reduced range of motion, and increasing debility. As a result, it is considered a leading cause of disability in the United States and has become a central public health concern.[3] OA affects approximately 20 million Americans, and the prevalence is predicted to double in the next 20 years.[4] There is more to the pathogenesis of OA than normal aging; factors including genetics, sex, age, obesity, joint trauma, and muscle strength play a part in disease pathogenesis.[2] Other mechanical aspects, such as joint instability and repetitive microtrauma, have also been implicated in perpetuating the disease process.[5] Medical therapy, including weight management and physical therapy, has primarily been directed toward the treatment of joint pain related to OA. Analgesics (acetaminophen, paracetamol) and nonsteroidal anti-inflammatory drugs (NSAIDs) are mainstream agents used in the treatment of OA-related pain. However, simple analgesics may be less effective than NSAIDs in short-term pain control.[6] Additionally, some studies have indicated that efficacy of NSAIDs for pain relief, including cyclooxygenase-2 inhibitors, is modest and can be associated with an increased risk of adverse events when used long-term.[7,8]

The authors have nothing to disclose.

[a] Division of Rheumatology, University of Utah School of Medicine, 30 North 1900 East, Salt Lake City, UT 84132, USA

[b] George E. Wahlen Department of Veterans Affairs Medical Center, 500 Foothill Drive, Salt Lake City, UT 84148, USA

* Corresponding author.

E-mail address: Karla.Miller@hsc.utah.edu

doi:10.1016/j.rdc.2010.11.007
0889-857X/11/$ – see front matter © 2011 Elsevier Inc. All rights reserved.
rheumatic.theclinics.com

Because available medical treatments for OA are modestly effective, at best, and most are directed at short-term pain control, the development of interventions that could relieve pain and potentially modify structural damage is very appealing. Substantial interest in glucosamine and chondroitin sulfate (often framed in lay literature as "cartilage precursors") abounds regarding the potential efficacy of glucosamine and chondroitin sulfate alone or in combination. Both of these agents are sold in the United States as dietary supplements and, therefore, are not required to meet the same safety and efficacy thresholds as drugs before they are approved to be marketed. Studies demonstrating efficacy of either agent alone or in combination have been of variable quality and have yielded inconsistent results. This article summarizes the current literature on these agents and their utility in the treatment of OA.

PREPARATIONS, BIOAVAILABILITY, AND PHARMACOKINETICS OF GLUCOSAMINE

Glucosamine is commercially available in a number of preparations. Some glucosamine preparations are extracted commercially by the acid hydrolysis of chitin derived from crustacean shells and, thus, patients with shellfish allergies should be advised to avoid the use of glucosamine manufactured in this manner. Because glucosamine is a weak organic base, it must be stabilized as a salt. The two most common and commercially available forms of oral glucosamine are in the form of glucosamine hydrochloride (HCl) and cocrystals or coprecipitates of glucosamine sulfate with potassium or sodium chloride.

Glucosamine HCl (**Fig. 1**A) is a very stable salt form of glucosamine that is available as a pure, oral preparation with a long shelf life. Hydrochloride salts are frequently used in combination with weak organic bases due to their favorable stability and solubility characteristics. Because of these characteristics, glucosamine HCl has been readily available for many years. The sulfate salt of glucosamine (see **Fig. 1**B) is extremely hygroscopic and readily deteriorates in ambient conditions making it impractical for oral ingestion. Over the years, methods to stabilize glucosamine hydrochloride as a cocrystal or coprecititate with either sodium chloride or potassium chloride were developed and patented that yielded a cocrystallized matrix of sodium chloride with glucosamine sulfate (see **Fig. 1**C). This product is suitable for oral dosing, and has subsequently been used in many commercially-sponsored OA trials.

Absolute daily dosing of glucosamine varies between and within various preparations due to the molecular size of the associated salt. Although no dosing studies have been conducted, recommended dosages of the final salt product generally range from 1250 mg to 1500 mg daily.

There are several studies that address the absorption, distribution, and metabolism of glucosamine. Glucosamine HCl given orally at clinically significant doses was shown to be bioavailable in both serum and synovium of horses and beagles.[9,10] Synovial concentrations of glucosamine remained elevated up to 12 hours, whereas

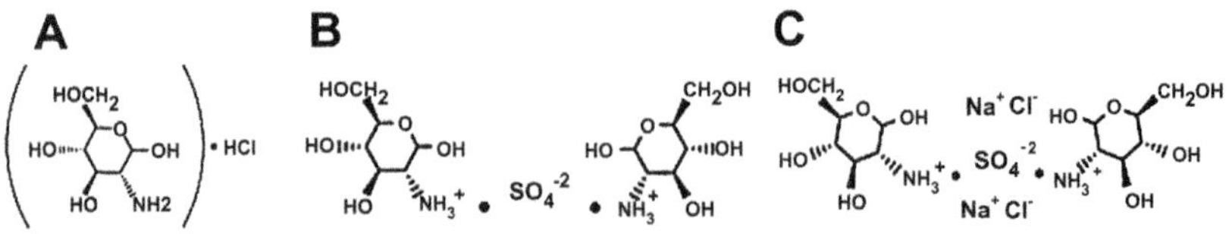

Fig. 1. Chemical structures of (A) glucosamine HCl, (B) glucosamine sulfate, and (C) glucosamine sulfate-sodium chloride coprecipitate.

serum levels were once again undetectable after 6 hours in the equine study.[9] Uptake of radiolabeled glucosamine sulfate by articular cartilage after oral dosing was shown in both rats and dogs.[11,12] These investigators also studied oral dosing in human volunteers.[13] Though absorption of radiolabeled oral glucosamine sulfate was 90%, there was a significant first-pass effect in the liver resulting in 44% bioavailability.[13] It is important to note that the specific methods for glucosamine detection in plasma were not sufficiently sensitive for monitoring its concentration in the unchanged form after oral dosing. A more recent study using liquid chromatography with mass spectrometry detection has been able to determine plasma concentrations more precisely, and has yielded an estimated half-life of 15 hours for oral-dose crystalline glucosamine sulfate.[14] This same study showed that glucosamine sulfate pharmacokinetics were linear up to the standard dosing of 1500 mg once daily, and higher doses did not result in a proportionally higher increase in glucosamine maximum concentration. Further animal studies have helped in determining an estimated bioavailability of 25%.[15] Interestingly, a recent human pharmacokinetic study revealed that combined dosing of glucosamine HCl with sodium chondroitin sulfate statistically significantly reduced circulating plasma levels of glucosamine compared with levels seen with glucosamine HCl dosed alone.[16]

PREPARATIONS, BIOAVAILABILITY, AND PHARMACOKINETICS OF CHONDROITIN SULFATE

Chondroitin 4-sulfate and chondroitin 6-sulfate are GAGs found in hyaline cartilage and differing structurally by the position of the monosaccharide that is sulfated (**Fig. 2**). They are very large, complex molecules. The position of chondroitin sulfation

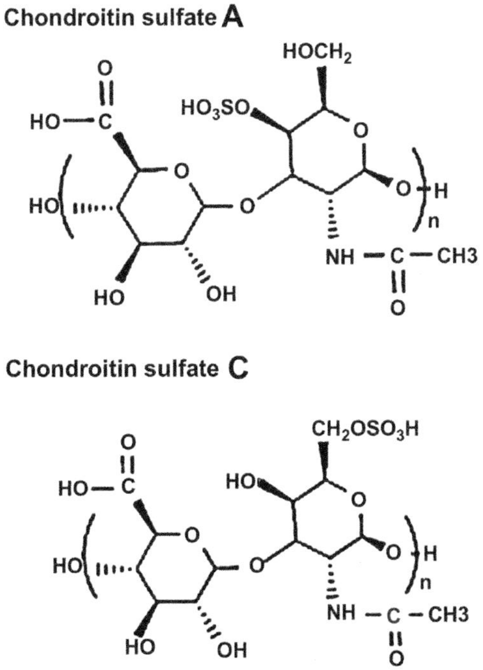

Fig. 2. Structure of chondroitin-4-sulfate A and chondroitin-6-sulfate C.

is of unclear significance but may be associated with aging tissue. Older, more superficial cartilage, contains higher proportions of chondroitin 6-sulfate, whereas newer, deeper cartilage, contains more chondroitin 4-sulfate.[17] In one study, ratios of chondroitin 6-sulfate to chondroitin 4-sulfate in cartilage affected by OA were substantially lower, but the clinical significance of this finding remains unclear.[18]

Sodium chondroitin sulfate is available in a number of oral preparations produced by multiple manufacturers. It is typically harvested from bovine and porcine tracheal cartilage, or occasionally from fish or avian cartilage. It is sold in the United States as a dietary supplement and does not require a prescription for purchase. The production process is not as strictly regulated as drugs, and differences in potency and quality are variable.[19,20] Although no formal dose finding studies have been conducted, commonly recommended dosages are between 800 and 1200 mg daily.

The oral bioavailability and pharmacokinetics of bovine-derived chondroitin sulfate were studied in healthy male volunteers by Volpi.[21] Plasma levels of chondroitin were monitored at regular intervals from baseline to 48 hours after oral administration of 4 g. Levels of chondroitin sulfate peaked at 2 hours and were increased by 200% at 2 to 4 hours. In a second study by the same investigator,[22] shark-derived chondroitin sulfate was administered instead, and similar peak plasma levels were documented at 8.7 hours. These observed discrepancies were attributed to the differences in molecular weights and charge densities of the two chondroitin sulfate molecules. Based on these studies and an additional study,[23] oral bioavailability of chondroitin sulfate is estimated at 5% to 15% with an elimination half-life of 6 hours and a range of peak plasma levels from 2 to 28 hours after administration. A recent publication on the human pharmacokinetics of clinically relevant doses of glucosamine HCl and sodium chondroitin sulfate could not detect a difference above circulating endogenous plasma levels of chondroitin sulfate after a single 1200 mg oral dose at all time periods from 0.25 to 36 hours.[16]

POSSIBLE MECHANISMS OF ACTION IN OSTEOARTHRITIS

Although there is conflicting evidence that orally supplemented glucosamine and chondroitin sulfate are bioavailable in the serum and synovial fluid, a defined mechanism of action by which they might alter the joint has not been demonstrated. The majority of in vitro studies addressing the effects of glucosamine on joints have been performed using concentrations of 50 to 5000 μM, which greatly exceeds the observed peak plasma concentration (Cmax) of 10 μM after clinically relevant glucosamine doses of 1500 mg per day in human studies.[24–27] Therefore, studies evaluating concentrations of glucosamine that are physiologically pertinent to the in vivo action of the drug are important for providing insight into possible mechanisms of action on joint tissues. One study evaluated incubated human chondrocytes affected by OA with glucosamine sulfate at concentrations ranging from 0.2 to 200 μM.[28] A significant increase in aggrecan core protein levels and its mRNA, as well as a reduction in matrix metalloproteinase-3, was noted at concentrations of glucosamine above 10 μM.[28] Another study looked at the effects of glucosamine HCl on equine chondrocytes and synoviocytes.[29] At concentrations of about 1 μM, glucosamine HCl appeared to interfere with interleukin-1 (IL-1) stimulation of prostaglandin E production in both types of cells.[29]

Relevant in vivo studies in rabbits and mice with papain-induced joint injury have shown increased cartilage GAG content after oral glucosamine administration.[30,31] One rabbit study used an anterior cruciate ligament deficient model of acute OA and daily oral administration of glucosamine HCl.[32] Glucosamine HCl was administered for 8 weeks starting at 3 weeks after surgery and no significant change in cartilage composition was noted, though there did seem to be a mild reduction in GAG loss from the femoral condyles.[32] A follow-up of this study observed that glucosamine HCl seemed to exert inhibitory effects on the bone turnover at the ligament resection site, noting the importance of studying all tissues pertaining to the joint rather than cartilage alone.[33]

The in vitro effects of chondroitin sulfate alone, and in combination with glucosamine, have also been studied. Some studies have shown a reduction in the expression of various proinflammatory enzymes and molecules such as phospholipase A2, cyclooxygenase-2, and prostaglandin E2.[34–36] One study found that the addition of chondroitin sulfate, in physiologic concentrations, to IL-1β-stimulated chondrocytes inhibited the nuclear translocation of nuclear factor-kappaB (NF-κB).[37] NF-κB is a transcription factor known to play a key role in the initiation of various proinflammatory genes involved in the pathogenesis of OA. Data addressing the in vivo activity of chondroitin sulfate is limited, but a few animal studies using chondroitin sulfate with or without glucosamine have been published. One study gave DBA/1 J mice with a type II collagen-induced arthritis varying dosages of chondroitin sulfate for 9 weeks and found a partial reduction in cartilage destruction, synovitis, and inflammatory cell infiltration.[38] It is important to note that these results were achieved at doses of 1000 mg/kg/d, which is significantly higher than typical doses taken by human subjects. Another study evaluated dogs previously treated with sodium chondroitin sulfate and glucosamine HCl who then underwent chymopapain injection of the radiocarpal joint to induce synovitis. This study indicated that prior treatment with sodium chondroitin sulfate resulted in less synovial inflammation.[39]

In light of the many in vitro studies, and a few in vivo studies, suggesting potential therapeutic effects for oral glucosamine and chondroitin sulfate, several clinical trials have sought to study the effects of these dietary supplements in human patients. Studying the effect of therapeutic interventions in OA has been complicated by many factors, including slow progression of the disease, increased placebo effect in larger trials,[40] use of agents of low therapeutic effect size, and difficulty in developing standardized outcome measures. In recent years, literature regarding the use of glucosamine and chondroitin sulfate alone, and in combination, for the treatment of OA has increased dramatically, yet clinical efficacy still remains controversial.

The surrogate markers for disease progression in clinical OA studies generally involve the assessment of pain and function or structural changes of the joint. The use of joint replacement as an endpoint for OA progression is complicated by the relatively small proportion of patients with OA that require this procedure, compared with the OA population at large. The two most common instruments used for measurement of pain and function in clinical OA trials are the Western Ontario and McMaster Universities Osteoarthritis (WOMAC) index[41] and the Lequesne index[42] questionnaires that base OA severity on parameters such as pain, stiffness, and functional activity.

Radiologic changes of OA are the most commonly used surrogate markers for disease progression. Most trials evaluating structural progression of OA assess knee joint space width (JSW) with formal measuring techniques. Though changes in JSW do not consistently correlate with symptoms of OA of the knee,[43] some studies have shown a correlation with knee arthroplasty.[44,45] There are a number of important issues that must be considered when obtaining measurements of JSW radiographically. Differences in positioning and weight-bearing can affect joint space measurements at the knee. For example, the presence of knee pain can alter JSW measurement, by limiting the degree of extension achieved.[46] The protocol published in 1996 by the Osteoarthritis Research Society International (OARSI) for knee imaging recommended weight-bearing anteroposterior (AP) fully extended knee views.[47]

However, subsequent studies[48–51] have shown superior reliability and sensitivity to change with detailed protocols that employ 20 to 30 degrees of knee flexion. Most trials have now incorporated the use of automated systems for JSW measurement from digital images as a way of minimizing error in measurement.

CLINICAL STUDIES OF GLUCOSAMINE IN OA
Symptoms

Some of the earlier clinical trials investigating the treatment of OA with glucosamine used a glucosamine sulfate preparation provided by the patent holder, Rottapharm.[52] These studies generally demonstrated a positive effect of glucosamine therapy on OA, but were fraught with shortcomings due to small sample size, inadequate allocation concealment, lack of intention-to-treat principles, and the propensity for sponsor bias. Subsequently, Rottapharm sponsored two larger, placebo-controlled studies that demonstrated a benefit of glucosamine sulfate treatment in both the symptoms and the radiographic progression of OA. The first study[53] evaluated 212 patients with knee OA over the 3 years and randomized one group to receive 1500 mg of oral glucosamine sulfate daily versus placebo. Though the primary outcome measure was radiographic progression, this study also looked at pain and function by WOMAC scores as percent change on a visual analog scale (VAS). This study found a statistically significant improvement in pain and function favoring glucosamine by WOMAC, but no improvement in stiffness. The second study[54] evaluated 202 similarly ascertained patients with knee OA using the same doses of glucosamine over 3 years. This study reported a significant change in WOMAC scores for pain, function, and stiffness in the glucosamine treated group. A comprehensive meta-analysis, published in 2005, reviewed the available literature on the efficacy of glucosamine monotherapy in the management of OA pain and function. This review by Towheed and colleagues[55] included nine trials using the Rotta preparation of glucosamine versus eight trials using non-Rotta preparations. Overall improvement in pain was noted with glucosamine versus placebo, and reported to be of clinical significance. However, results for efficacy in function were variable with significant changes reported for Lequesne index, but not for WOMAC total scores or subscores. Subgroup analysis in patients taking the Rotta glucosamine preparation demonstrated significant improvement in WOMAC total scores, but no significant change was reported in function outcomes for non-Rotta preparations. In the late 1990s, the National Institutes of Health (NIH) funded a large, double-blind, placebo- and celecoxib-controlled, multicenter clinical trial to more carefully evaluate the efficacy and safety of glucosamine and chondroitin sulfate alone and in combination in the treatment of OA of the knee. The Glucosamine/chondroitin Arthritis Intervention Trial[56] (GAIT) enrolled 1583 patients with symptomatic knee OA and randomized them to receive glucosamine HCl 1500 mg daily, sodium chondroitin sulfate 1200 mg daily, both in combination at the same daily doses, celecoxib 200 mg daily, or placebo for 24 weeks. The primary outcome measure was a 20% decrease in WOMAC Pain at 24 weeks compared with baseline. The results demonstrated that glucosamine was not significantly better than placebo in the overall reduction of knee pain. Glucosamine showed a trend toward significance in the subgroup of patients with moderate to severe knee pain treated with glucosamine, but interpretation of this result was limited by the small number of patients in this subgroup. A GAIT ancillary study recently published 2-year results on 662 patients with knee OA randomized to the same treatments, and found no clinically important improvement in WOMAC pain or function compared with placebo.[8] Although the glucosamine and celecoxib groups showed beneficial trends for pain and function, they did not reach statistical significance.

Structural Modification

The placebo-controlled studies evaluating the long-term effects of glucosamine on structural progression of knee OA are limited; three studies of reasonable quality evaluated glucosamine with a primary outcome of change in JSW. The results of the pain and function secondary outcome measures of two of these studies are reviewed above, and the third study was a GAIT ancillary study published in 2008.[57] The first study[53] evaluated 212 patients with knee OA for radiographic progression. Patients were randomized to receive 1500 mg of glucosamine sulfate daily versus placebo over 3 years. Standing, weight-bearing, AP knee radiographs were obtained sequentially to determine change in medial compartment JSW. The investigators noted progressive cartilage loss in patients receiving placebo and no joint space loss in patients taking glucosamine sulfate. The second study[54] evaluated 202 patients randomized similarly and using the same radiographic techniques as the first study, and also found no joint space loss in the glucosamine group compared with the placebo group. The third study[57] was a 24-month GAIT ancillary study that enrolled 572 patients with radiographic OA of the knees and randomized them to receive glucosamine HCl, sodium chondroitin sulfate, the combination of both, celecoxib, and placebo in the doses described earlier for GAIT. Radiographic data were obtained using the metatarsophalangeal (MTP) radiographic view of the knee joints at 12 and 24 months. No statistically significant difference in mean JSW measured at the medial tibiofemoral joint was observed for any group compared with placebo, though there was a trend toward improvement in patients with milder OA receiving glucosamine. One notable difference between the first two studies and the third study was the use of different imaging techniques. The first two studies obtained their measurements of JSW from AP extended views of the knee, whereas the third study used the semi-flexed MTP view described by Buckland-Wright and colleagues.[48] JSWmeasured on extended AP views may measure other structures such as the menisci and collateral ligaments, and not only articular cartilage. Additionally, the presence of joint pain at the time of imaging may alter the ability to achieve full extension, thereby giving the appearance of reduced JSW.[46]

CLINICAL STUDIES OF CHONDROITIN SULFATE IN OA
Symptoms

Efficacy of chondroitin sulfate over placebo for treating pain in OA was reported in many of the smaller, earlier studies, but the estimates varied considerably from study to study. In recent years, larger-scale trials have reported little to no effect of chondroitin sulfate treatment on the symptoms of OA. GAIT was designed to rigorously assess the efficacy of glucosamine and chondroitin sulfate in symptomatic knee OA, and failed to find any statistically significantly greater efficacy of either of these agents alone, or in combination, than that of placebo.[56] Interestingly, a post hoc analysis of the GAIT demonstrated a potential benefit of chondroitin sulfate treatment on joint swelling in the subgroup of patients with earlier OA.[58] Reichenbach and colleagues[59] published a meta-analysis evaluating the effect of chondroitin sulfate on pain related to knee or hip OA as the primary objective. The investigators found substantial heterogeneity among trials, rendering the interpretation of results challenging. They subsequently pooled the three trials with larger sample sizes, intention-to-treat analyses, and adequate allocation concealment, and found chondroitin sulfate to be ineffective for symptom management in these trials. Another meta-analysis published the same year assessed randomized controlled trial (RCT) data on various analgesic agents for short-term management of pain in OA.[60] A total of 362 patients from six RCTs provided data on chondroitin sulfate, and a small statistically significant benefit in pain relief was noted at 4 weeks. However, the observed effects were smaller than the thresholds for clinically relevant improvement. A recent RCT evaluating chondroitin sulfate in structural progression of knee OA in 662 patients studied pain as a secondary outcome measure over 2 years and found more rapid improvement in pain by VAS and WOMAC, though statistical significance did not persist after 9 months.[61] The results of a 2-year ancillary GAIT study were published recently, and no clinically important difference in WOMAC pain or function was detected for any treatment, including chondroitin sulfate alone or in combination.[8]

Structural Modification

As discussed above, data regarding modification of pain and function in OA do not consistently correlate to changes in JSW, and this is especially evident in studies of chondroitin sulfate. In the meta-analysis published by Reichenbach and colleagues,[59] results on JSW were evaluated as a secondary objective. Five of the 20 studies included in the analysis evaluated JSW and, though small effect on joint space narrowing (JSN) in favor of chondroitin sulfate was noted, it was of uncertain clinical significance. The GAIT ancillary study published in 2008 reported 2-year data on knee OA progression with chondroitin sulfate alone and in combination with glucosamine.[57] No significant difference in mean loss of JSW at 2 years was observed in any of the treatment groups compared with placebo. The investigators noted limitation of the study due to limited sample size, variance in JSW measurement, and smaller than expected JSW loss. Interestingly, the loss in JSW in the treatment group receiving glucosamine and chondroitin sulfate was greater than in patients treated with glucosamine or chondroitin sulfate alone. Subsequently, the Study on Osteoarthritis Progression Prevention published results on the effects of chondroitins 4 and 6 sulfate on minimum JSW loss over 2 years.[61] Minimum JSW loss was the primary outcome measure and the study randomized 622 patients to receive chondroitin sulfate 800 mg or placebo daily. A significant reduction in minimum JSW loss was reported in the chondroitin sulfate group compared with placebo, though the clinical importance of this reduction remains unclear.

CLINICAL STUDIES OF GLUCOSAMINE IN COMBINATION WITH CHONDROITIN SULFATE IN OA
Symptoms

Fewer data have been published on the combination glucosamine and chondroitin sulfate product than on either agent alone, though they are commonly available and taken as a combination supplement. GAIT was the largest and most rigorous study that evaluated the effects of glucosamine HCl and sodium chondroitin sulfate in combination compared with placebo over 24 weeks.[56] These agents alone or in combination did not reduce pain effectively in patients with knee OA overall, but exploratory analysis suggested a potential benefit of the combination in patients with moderate-to-severe knee pain. There was no significant difference in secondary outcomes, such as stiffness, VAS, and function measures, for glucosamine HCl, sodium chondroitin sulfate, or the combination compared with placebo. Additionally, 2-year results from GAIT published recently indicated no clinically significant difference in WOMAC pain or function compared with placebo, though glucosamine and celecoxib showed beneficial trends.[8] Other, less rigorous studies have evaluated combination glucosamine and chondroitin sulfate compared with placebo.

Messier and colleagues[62] evaluated the effects of glucosamine 1500 mg plus chondroitin sulfate 1200 mg per day with exercise versus placebo with exercise on function in 89 patients with knee OA over the course of 12 months. This study failed to identify any difference in function, mobility, and pain in those taking the combination supplement compared with placebo, regardless of the addition of exercise to both groups in the last 6 months of the study. A study by Rai[63] in 2004 evaluated efficacy of glucosamine sulfate 250 mg daily and sodium chondroitin sulfate 200 mg daily in 100 patients compared with placebo with a primary outcome measure of change in minimum JSW and a secondary outcome of pain or function as assessed by Lequesne Index over 12 months. The investigator reported a significant improvement in Lequesne Index scores in the intervention group as compared with placebo. However, this study did not discuss randomization methods, allocation concealment, or analysis.

Structural Modification

The study by Rai[63] also evaluated change in minimum JSW as the primary outcome. The study reported a statistically significant difference for preservation of minimum JSW in the intervention group when compared with placebo. This study did not report on method of randomization, allocation concealment, and intention-to-treat analyses, making interpretation of the results challenging. The GAIT ancillary study on structural progression in knee OA reported data on combined glucosamine HCl and sodium chondroitin sulfate and found no clinically important differences in JSW loss compared with placebo.[57]

OTHER STUDIES

Most data regarding the use of glucosamine and chondroitin sulfate in the treatment of OA deals with the knee joint. Two studies published in recent years evaluated the effects of glucosamine sulfate on pain, function, and radiographic progression of OA in the hip. The first study[64] randomized 222 patients with hip OA to receive either 1500 mg of glucosamine sulfate daily or placebo over 24 months. They noted no difference in WOMAC pain or function subscores, and no difference in JSN between the two groups. Additionally, a subgroup analysis of this study evaluated results by OA severity and presence of generalized or diffuse disease.[65] Again, no significant differences were identified in regard to pain, function, or JSN between glucosamine and placebo treated subgroups. One recently published study evaluated the use of glucosamine in patients with chronic low back pain and degenerative lumbar OA.[66] The study randomized 250 patients to receive glucosamine 1500 mg daily or placebo over 12 months. Pain-related disability assessed by questionnaire was the primary outcome measure and no significant difference in outcome was observed at 6 or 12 months. There are very limited data addressing the use of glucosamine or chondroitin sulfate in OA of the hands.

SAFETY

Long-term clinical data regarding the safety of glucosamine and chondroitin sulfate alone, or in combination, is limited. However, none of the trials or systematic reviews discussed thus far found significant differences in reported adverse effects compared with placebo, including studies of 2 to 3 years in duration. Importantly, some trials did not report systematically on adverse effects.

Glucosamine

One concern specific to glucosamine is the potential risk of diabetes onset or worsening because animal studies have shown an association between increased intracellular glucosamine and insulin resistance.[67–69] Two nonsystematic reviews evaluated the effects of glucosamine on serum glucose levels, and found no significant changes in serum glucose levels compared with placebo with therapeutic dosing of glucosamine.[70,71] Additionally, the 3-year studies by Pavelka[54] and Reginster[53] found no significant change in glucose levels between the two groups, though their data was limited. Scroggie and colleagues[72] evaluated hemoglobin A1c levels in 34 patients with type 2 diabetes mellitus given daily glucosamine 1500 mg and sodium chondroitin sulfate 1200 mg after 90 days. They found no significant differences in the intervention group compared with placebo.

Chondroitin Sulfate

As mentioned earlier, chondroitin sulfate is well-tolerated and without significant adverse effects above placebo. One particular safety concern with chondroitin sulfate is the possibility for bovine spongiform encephalopathy (mad cow disease) transmission from infected products derived from beef. Though no cases of this disease have been reported in association with taking chondroitin sulfate supplements, there has been a case reported in an American herd, raising the question of potential risk. Patients who take chondroitin sulfate should be aware of this possibility, and confirm that the supplement is derived from a disease-free animal source.

Glucosamine and Chondroitin Sulfate

A case report[73] published in 2008 reported a potential glucosamine-chondroitin sulfate and warfarin interaction in a patient resulting in an increased international normalized ratio (INR). This resulted in a search of multiple databases for increased INR in patients taking glucosamine or glucosamine-chondroitin sulfate supplements. Forty-three cases of increased INR were identified, and some of the reports documented a stable INR before initiation of the supplement and resolution to a stable INR once the supplement was stopped. In light of the potential risk of bleeding associated with an increased INR, the investigators recommended cautious use of these supplements or avoidance in patients on warfarin therapy.

DISCUSSION

In reviewing OA trials, it is important to note that trials developed to evaluate structural progression may not be adequately designed for detecting differences in pain and function. In addition, slowing of radiographic progression may not correlate with relief of symptoms, raising concern about the clinical importance of these findings. OA is a slowly progressive disease, and evidence of disease modification with an intervention may not be apparent for many years.

A recent systematic review published by Black and colleagues[74] in the United Kingdom assessed the clinical effectiveness of glucosamine, chondroitin sulfate, and the combination on both symptoms and structural progression of knee OA, as well as performed a cost analysis based on available data. The investigators concluded that some evidence of long-term effectiveness for the Rotta preparation of glucosamine sulfate exists. They found evidence of effectiveness for glucosamine HCl, sodium chondroitin sulfate, and the combination of glucosamine HCl-sulfate with chondroitin sulfate to be lacking, largely due to heterogeneity in trial results.

Interestingly, a cost analysis of glucosamine sulfate in treatment of knee OA did not convincingly support cost-effectiveness.

Considerable discrepancy between clinical efficacy of glucosamine sulfate and glucosamine HCl is apparent in the literature and favors glucosamine sulfate. Some studies have suggested that differences between these preparations could be explained on the basis of the sulfate anion.[75–77] The proposed mechanism suggests that the sulfate anion in the circulation is limiting on chondroitin synthesis, and supplements containing the sulfate anion may therefore increase synthesis of chondroitin sulfate.[78,79] Others have indicated that routine dosing of oral glucosamine sulfate would have to increase the serum sulfate 50-fold to have a substantial effect on the sulfate supply.[80] It is important to note that, once ingested, either glucosamine salt form readily dissociates and is absorbed as glucosamine. Thus, regardless of the salt form, in pharmacokinetic studies, only the glucosamine is measured in the serum.[11–13] Additionally,[14]C-radiolabeled glucosamine hydrochloride mixed with unlabeled cocrystallized glucosamine sulfate was used in these early pharmacokinetic studies.[11–13] It is still uncertain whether a genuine difference exists between glucosamine sulfate and glucosamine HCl preparations, or whether the apparent heterogeneity among trials is a result of inadequate concealment and industry bias.[81] Conclusive evidence supporting the superiority of cocrystallized glucosamine sulfate over glucosamine HCl on the basis of glucosamine as the active ingredient has not been published.

Glucosamine and chondroitin sulfate are dietary supplements that are also found naturally in the body. The best current evidence suggests that the effect of these supplements, alone or in combination, on OA pain, function, and radiographic change is marginal at best.[82] The cost-effectiveness of these dietary supplements alone or in combination in the treatment of OA has not been demonstrated in North America. Some patients take these supplements due to a perceived benefit that could represent placebo response, variable absorption, or actual differences in preparations. Despite the lack of efficacy reported in many trials, consumer behavior regarding the use of oral supplements continues unaltered and further research aimed at clarifying current evidence may not impact public behavior.[83] Nevertheless, data from many trials to date support a benign safety profile for all of these supplements, and patients who desire to take them can be reassured that dangerous adverse effects are unlikely, though caution should be advised in patients taking concurrent warfarin.

REFERENCES

1. Wollheim FA. Pathogenesis of osteoarthritis. In: Hochberg MC, Silman AJ, Smolen JS, et al, editors. Rheumatology, vol. 2. 3rd edition. Edinburgh (UK), London, New York, Philadelphia, St Louis, Sydney, Toronto: Mosby; 2003. p. 1801.
2. Felson DT, Lawrence RC, Dieppe PA, et al. Osteoarthritis: new insights. Part 1: the disease and its risk factors. Ann Intern Med 2000;133:635.
3. McNeil JM, Binette J. Centers for Disease Control and Prevention: prevalence of disabilities and associated health conditions among adults–United States, 1999. MMWR Morb Mortal Wkly Rep 2001;50:101.
4. Lawrence RC, Felson DT, Helmick CG, et al. Estimates of the prevalence of arthritis and other rheumatic conditions in the United States. Part II. Arthritis Rheum 2008;58:26.
5. Brandt KD, Radin EL, Dieppe PA, et al. Yet more evidence that osteoarthritis is not a cartilage disease. Ann Rheum Dis 2006;65:1261.

6. Towheed TE, Maxwell L, Judd MG, et al. Acetaminophen for osteoarthritis. Cochrane Database Syst Rev 2006;1:CD004257.
7. Rostom A, Muir K, Dube C, et al. Gastrointestinal safety of cyclooxygenase-2 inhibitors: a Cochrane Collaboration systematic review. Clin Gastroenterol Hepatol 2007;5:818.
8. Sawitzke AD, Shi H, Finco MF, et al. Clinical efficacy and safety of glucosamine, chondroitin sulphate, their combination, celecoxib or placebo taken to treat osteoarthritis of the knee: 2-year results from GAIT. Ann Rheum Dis 2010;69:1459–64.
9. Laverty S, Sandy JD, Celeste C, et al. Synovial fluid levels and serum pharmacokinetics in a large animal model following treatment with oral glucosamine at clinically relevant doses. Arthritis Rheum 2005;52:181.
10. Adebowale A, Du J, Liang Z, et al. The bioavailability and pharmacokinetics of glucosamine hydrochloride and low molecular weight chondroitin sulfate after single and multiple doses to beagle dogs. Biopharm Drug Dispos 2002;23:217.
11. Setnikar I, Giacchetti C, Zanolo G. Pharmacokinetics of glucosamine in the dog and in man. Arzneimittelforschung 1986;36:729.
12. Setnikar I, Giachetti C, Zanolo G. Absorption, distribution and excretion of radioactivity after a single intravenous or oral administration of [14C] glucosamine to the rat. Pharmatherapeutica 1984;3:538.
13. Setnikar I, Palumbo R, Canali S, et al. Pharmacokinetics of glucosamine in man. Arzneimittelforschung 1993;43:1109.
14. Persiani S, Roda E, Rovati LC, et al. Glucosamine oral bioavailability and plasma pharmacokinetics after increasing doses of crystalline glucosamine sulfate in man. Osteoarthritis Cartilage 2005;13:1041.
15. Persiani S, Locatelli M, Fiorentino S, et al. Absolute bioavailability of glucosamine after administration of crystalline glucosamine sulfate in rats. Osteoarthritis Cartilage 2005;13(Suppl A):P161.
16. Jackson CG, Plaas AH, Sandy JD, et al. The human pharmacokinetics of oral ingestion of glucosamine and chondroitin sulfate taken separately or in combination. Osteoarthritis Cartilage 2010;18:297.
17. Bayliss MT, Osborne D, Woodhouse S, et al. Sulfation of chondroitin sulfate in human articular cartilage. The effect of age, topographical position, and zone of cartilage on tissue composition. J Biol Chem 1999;274:15892.
18. Burkhardt D, Michel BA, Baici A, et al. Comparison of chondroitin sulphate composition of femoral head articular cartilage from patients with femoral neck fractures and osteoarthritis and controls. Rheumatol Int 1995;14:235.
19. Barnhill JG, Fye CL, Williams DW, et al. Chondroitin product selection for the glucosamine/chondroitin arthritis intervention trial. J Am Pharm Assoc 2006; 46:14.
20. Joint remedies. Consum Rep 2002;67:18–21.
21. Volpi N. Oral bioavailability of chondroitin sulfate (Condrosulf) and its constituents in healthy male volunteers. Osteoarthritis Cartilage 2002;10:768.
22. Volpi N. Oral absorption and bioavailability of ichthyic origin chondroitin sulfate in healthy male volunteers. Osteoarthritis Cartilage 2003;11:433.
23. Conte A, Volpi N, Palmieri L, et al. Biochemical and pharmacokinetic aspects of oral treatment with chondroitin sulfate. Arzneimittelforschung 1995;45:918.
24. Huang TM, Cai L, Yang B, et al. Liquid chromatography with electrospray ionization mass spectrometry method for the assay of glucosamine sulfate in human plasma: validation and application to a pharmacokinetic study. Biomed Chromatogr 2006;20:251.

25. Roda A, Sabatini L, Barbieri A, et al. Development and validation of a sensitive HPLC-ESI-MS/MS method for the direct determination of glucosamine in human plasma. J Chromatogr B Analyt Technol Biomed Life Sci 2006;844:119.
26. Zhang LJ, Huang TM, Fang XL, et al. Determination of glucosamine sulfate in human plasma by precolumn derivatization using high performance liquid chromatography with fluorescence detection: its application to a bioequivalence study. J Chromatogr B Analyt Technol Biomed Life Sci 2006;842:8.
27. Zhong S, Zhong D, Chen X. Improved and simplified liquid chromatography/electrospray ionization mass spectrometry method for the analysis of underivatized glucosamine in human plasma. J Chromatogr B Analyt Technol Biomed Life Sci 2007;854:291.
28. Dodge GR, Jimenez SA. Glucosamine sulfate modulates the levels of aggrecan and matrix metalloproteinase-3 synthesized by cultured human osteoarthritis articular chondrocytes. Osteoarthritis Cartilage 2003;11:424.
29. Byron CRSM, Stewart AA, Pondenis HC. Effects of clinically relevant concentrations of glucosamine on equine chondrocytes and synoviocytes in vitro. Am J Vet Res 2008;69:1129.
30. Oegema TR Jr, Deloria LB, Sandy JD, et al. Effect of oral glucosamine on cartilage and meniscus in normal and chymopapain-injected knees of young rabbits. Arthritis Rheum 2002;46:2495.
31. Panicker S, Borgia J, Fhied C, et al. Oral glucosamine modulates the response of the liver and lymphocytes of the mesenteric lymph nodes in a papain-induced model of joint damage and repair. Osteoarthritis Cartilage 2009;17:1014.
32. Tiraloche G, Girard C, Chouinard L, et al. Effect of oral glucosamine on cartilage degradation in a rabbit model of osteoarthritis. Arthritis Rheum 2005;52:1118.
33. Wang SX, Laverty S, Dumitriu M, et al. The effects of glucosamine hydrochloride on subchondral bone changes in an animal model of osteoarthritis. Arthritis Rheum 2007;56:1537.
34. Chan PS, Caron JP, Orth MW. Effect of glucosamine and chondroitin sulfate on regulation of gene expression of proteolytic enzymes and their inhibitors in interleukin-1-challenged bovine articular cartilage explants. Am J Vet Res 1870;66:2005.
35. Orth MW, Peters TL, Hawkins JN. Inhibition of articular cartilage degradation by glucosamine-HCl and chondroitin sulphate. Equine Vet J Suppl 2002;(34):224.
36. Ronca F, Palmieri L, Panicucci P, et al. Anti-inflammatory activity of chondroitin sulfate. Osteoarthritis Cartilage 1998;6(Suppl A):14.
37. Jomphe C, Gabriac M, Hale TM, et al. Chondroitin sulfate inhibits the nuclear translocation of nuclear factor-kappaB in interleukin-1beta-stimulated chondrocytes. Basic Clin Pharmacol Toxicol 2008;102:59.
38. Omata T, Itokazu Y, Inoue N, et al. Effects of chondroitin sulfate-C on articular cartilage destruction in murine collagen-induced arthritis. Arzneimittelforschung 2000;50:148.
39. Canapp SO Jr, McLaughlin RM Jr, Hoskinson JJ, et al. Scintigraphic evaluation of dogs with acute synovitis after treatment with glucosamine hydrochloride and chondroitin sulfate. Am J Vet Res 1999;60:1552.
40. Zhang W, Robertson J, Jones AC, et al. The placebo effect and its determinants in osteoarthritis: meta-analysis of randomised controlled trials. Ann Rheum Dis 2008;67:1716.
41. Bellamy N, Buchanan WW, Goldsmith CH, et al. Validation study of WOMAC: a health status instrument for measuring clinically important patient relevant

outcomes to antirheumatic drug therapy in patients with osteoarthritis of the hip or knee. J Rheumatol 1833;15:1988.

42. Lequesne M. Indices of severity and disease activity for osteoarthritis. Semin Arthritis Rheum 1991;20:48.

43. Dieppe PA, Cushnaghan J, Shepstone L. The Bristol 'OA500' study: progression of osteoarthritis (OA) over 3 years and the relationship between clinical and radiographic changes at the knee joint. Osteoarthritis Cartilage 1997;5:87.

44. Bruyere O, Pavelka K, Rovati LC, et al. Total joint replacement after glucosamine sulphate treatment in knee osteoarthritis: results of a mean 8-year observation of patients from two previous 3-year, randomised, placebo-controlled trials. Osteoarthritis Cartilage 2008;16:254.

45. Cicuttini FM, Jones G, Forbes A, et al. Rate of cartilage loss at two years predicts subsequent total knee arthroplasty: a prospective study. Ann Rheum Dis 2004;63: 1124.

46. Mazzuca SA, Brandt KD, Lane KA, et al. Knee pain reduces joint space width in conventional standing anteroposterior radiographs of osteoarthritic knees. Arthritis Rheum 2002;46:1223.

47. Altman R, Brandt K, Hochberg M, et al. Design and conduct of clinical trials in patients with osteoarthritis: recommendations from a task force of the Osteoarthritis Research Society. Results from a workshop. Osteoarthritis Cartilage 1996;4:217.

48. Buckland-Wright JC, Wolfe F, Ward RJ, et al. Substantial superiority of semiflexed (MTP) views in knee osteoarthritis: a comparative radiographic study, without fluoroscopy, of standing extended, semiflexed (MTP), and schuss views. J Rheumatol 1999;26:2664.

49. Peterfy C, Li J, Zaim S, et al. Comparison of fixed-flexion positioning with fluoroscopic semi-flexed positioning for quantifying radiographic joint-space width in the knee: test-retest reproducibility. Skeletal Radiol 2003;32:128.

50. Piperno M, Hellio Le Graverand MP, Conrozier T, et al. Quantitative evaluation of joint space width in femorotibial osteoarthritis: comparison of three radiographic views. Osteoarthritis Cartilage 1998;6:252.

51. Vignon E, Piperno M, Le Graverand MP, et al. Measurement of radiographic joint space width in the tibiofemoral compartment of the osteoarthritic knee: comparison of standing anteroposterior and Lyon schuss views. Arthritis Rheum 2003;48:378.

52. McAlindon TE, LaValley MP, Felson DT. Efficacy of glucosamine and chondroitin for treatment of osteoarthritis. JAMA 2000;284:1241.

53. Reginster JY, Deroisy R, Rovati LC, et al. Long-term effects of glucosamine sulphate on osteoarthritis progression: a randomised, placebo-controlled clinical trial. Lancet 2001;357:251.

54. Pavelka K, Gatterova J, Olejarova M, et al. Glucosamine sulfate use and delay of progression of knee osteoarthritis: a 3-year, randomized, placebo-controlled, double-blind study. Arch Intern Med 2002;162:2113.

55. Towheed TE, Maxwell L, Anastassiades TP, et al. Glucosamine therapy for treating osteoarthritis. Cochrane Database Syst Rev 2005;2:CD002946.

56. Clegg DO, Reda DJ, Harris CL, et al. Glucosamine, chondroitin sulfate and the two in combination for painful knee osteoarthritis. N Engl J Med 2006;354:795–808.

57. Sawitzke AD, Shi H, Finco MF, et al. The effect of glucosamine and/or chondroitin sulfate on the progression of knee osteoarthritis: a report from the glucosamine/chondroitin arthritis intervention trial. Arthritis Rheum 2008;58:3183.

58. Hochberg MC, Clegg DO. Potential effects of chondroitin sulfate on joint swelling: a GAIT report. Osteoarthritis Cartilage 2008;16(Suppl 3):S22.

59. Reichenbach S, Sterchi R, Scherer M, et al. Meta-analysis: chondroitin for osteoarthritis of the knee or hip. Ann Intern Med 2007;146:580.
60. Bjordal JM, Klovning A, Ljunggren AE, et al. Short-term efficacy of pharmacotherapeutic interventions in osteoarthritic knee pain: a meta-analysis of randomised placebo-controlled trials. Eur J Pain 2007;11:125.
61. Kahan A, Uebelhart D, De Vathaire F, et al. Long-term effects of chondroitins 4 and 6 sulfate on knee osteoarthritis: the study on osteoarthritis progression prevention, a two-year, randomized, double-blind, placebo-controlled trial. Arthritis Rheum 2009;60:524.
62. Messier SP, Mihalko S, Loeser RF, et al. Glucosamine/chondroitin combined with exercise for the treatment of knee osteoarthritis: a preliminary study. Osteoarthritis Cartilage 2007;15:1256.
63. Rai J. Efficacy of chondroitin sulfate and glucosamine sulfate in the progression of symptomatic knee osteoarthritis: a randomized, placebo-controlled, double-blind study. Bull Postgrad Inst Med Educ Res Chandigarh 2004;38:18.
64. Rozendaal RM, Koes BW, van Osch GJ, et al. Effect of glucosamine sulfate on hip osteoarthritis: a randomized trial. Ann Intern Med 2008;148:268.
65. Rozendaal RM, Uitterlinden EJ, van Osch GJ, et al. Effect of glucosamine sulphate on joint space narrowing, pain and function in patients with hip osteoarthritis; subgroup analyses of a randomized controlled trial. Osteoarthritis Cartilage 2009;17:427.
66. Wilkens P, Scheel IB, Grundnes O, et al. Effect of glucosamine on pain-related disability in patients with chronic low back pain and degenerative lumbar osteoarthritis: a randomized controlled trial. JAMA 2010;304:45.
67. McClain DA, Crook ED. Hexosamines and insulin resistance. Diabetes 1996;45:1003.
68. Rossetti L. Perspective: hexosamines and nutrient sensing. Endocrinology 1922;141:2000.
69. Tang J, Neidigh JL, Cooksey RC, et al. Transgenic mice with increased hexosamine flux specifically targeted to beta-cells exhibit hyperinsulinemia and peripheral insulin resistance. Diabetes 2000;49:1492.
70. Anderson JW, Nicolosi RJ, Borzelleca JF. Glucosamine effects in humans: a review of effects on glucose metabolism, side effects, safety considerations and efficacy. Food Chem Toxicol 2005;43:187.
71. Stumpf JL, Lin SW. Effect of glucosamine on glucose control. Ann Pharmacother 2006;40:694.
72. Scroggie DA, Albright A, Harris MD. The effect of glucosamine-chondroitin supplementation on glycosylated hemoglobin levels in patients with type 2 diabetes mellitus: a placebo-controlled, double-blinded, randomized clinical trial. Arch Intern Med 2003;163:1587.
73. Knudsen JF, Sokol GH. Potential glucosamine-warfarin interaction resulting in increased international normalized ratio: case report and review of the literature and MedWatch database. Pharmacotherapy 2008;28:540.
74. Black C, Clar C, Henderson R, et al. The clinical effectiveness of glucosamine and chondroitin supplements in slowing or arresting progression of osteoarthritis of the knee: a systematic review and economic evaluation. Health Technol Assess 2009;13:1.
75. Ikeda T, Mabuchi A, Fukuda A, et al. Identification of sequence polymorphisms in two sulfation-related genes, PAPSS2 and SLC26A2, and an association analysis with knee osteoarthritis. J Hum Genet 2001;46:538.
76. Silbert JE. Dietary glucosamine under question. Glycobiology 2009;19:564.

77. Uldry M, Ibberson M, Hosokawa M, et al. GLUT2 is a high affinity glucosamine transporter. FEBS Lett 2002;524:199.
78. Blinn CM, Dibbs ER, Hronowski LJ, et al. Fasting serum sulfate levels before and after development of osteoarthritis in participants of the veterans administration normative aging longitudinal study do not differ from levels in participants in whom osteoarthritis did not develop. Arthritis Rheum 2005;52:2808.
79. Cordoba F, Nimni ME. Chondroitin sulfate and other sulfate containing chondro-protective agents may exhibit their effects by overcoming a deficiency of sulfur amino acids. Osteoarthritis Cartilage 2003;11:228.
80. Block JA, Oegema TR, Sandy JD, et al. The effects of oral glucosamine on joint health: is a change in research approach needed? Osteoarthritis Cartilage 2010; 18:5.
81. Vlad SC, LaValley MP, McAlindon TE, et al. Glucosamine for pain in osteoarthritis: why do trial results differ? Arthritis Rheum 2007;56:2267.
82. Wandel S, Juni P, Tendal B, et al. Effects of glucosamine, chondroitin, or placebo in patients with osteoarthritis of hip or knee: network meta-analysis. BMJ 2010; 341:c4675.
83. Tilburt J, Emanuel EJ, Miller FG. Does the evidence make a difference in consumer behavior? Sales of supplements before and after publication of negative research results. J Gen Intern Med 2008;23:1495.

Role of Diet in Rheumatic Disease

Sophia Li, MD[a],*, Robert Micheletti, MD[b]

KEYWORDS

- Diet • Nutrition • Gout • Fibromyalgia • Osteoarthritis
- Rheumatoid arthritis

Millions of people suffer from rheumatic diseases. This article reviews available research on the effects of diet on these diseases.

GOUT AND DIET

Gout is an inflammatory arthritis associated with hyperuricemia and caused by the precipitation of monosodium urate crystals in joints and soft tissues. It has been linked to components of the metabolic syndrome—hypertension, obesity, diabetes mellitus, and hyperlipidemia—as well as to consumption of purine-rich food and drink. Whereas prospective studies confirming these associations were previously lacking, there is now sufficient evidence to support lifestyle and dietary modification as a means of preventing gout.

Purine-Rich Foods

Diets high in protein and alcohol have long been thought to increase the risk of gout. Metabolic studies have shown that increased purified purine loads can raise serum uric acid concentration.[1] For this reason, patients with gout have traditionally been encouraged to adhere to severely purine-restricted diets. Such diets can decrease the serum urate concentration by about 1 mg/dL but may be too impractical or unpalatable for long-term adherence.[2,3] Conversely, modifications like those recommended for patients with insulin resistance, emphasizing caloric restriction and avoidance of saturated fat and refined carbohydrates, may be more palatable and have shown the ability both to decrease serum urate and to diminish the recurrence of gout. In a group of 13 men on such a diet, serum urate levels dropped an average of 1.7 mg/dL, and the number of monthly gout attacks decreased from 2.1 to 0.6. Weight loss and improved lipid profiles were other benefits.[4]

a Division of Rheumatology, Department of Medicine, University of Pennsylvania, 3400 Spruce Street, Philadelphia, PA 19104, USA
b Department of Medicine, University of Pennsylvania, 100 Centrex, 3400 Spruce Street, Philadelphia, PA 19104, USA
* Corresponding author.
E-mail address: sophia.li@uphs.upenn.edu

Rheum Dis Clin N Am 37 (2011) 119–133
doi:10.1016/j.rdc.2010.11.006
0889-857X/11/$ – see front matter © 2011 Elsevier Inc. All rights reserved.

These findings suggest dietary modification might be of value in preventing gout attacks but are limited by the small number of subjects and lack of data on specific foods. To elucidate the relationship between dietary risk factors and incident gout in more detail, the Health Professionals Follow-up Study (HPFS) followed 47,150 men with no baseline history of gout prospectively for 12 years. In that span, there were 730 incident cases of gout. Men in the highest quintile of meat intake (namely beef, pork, and lamb) were 41% more likely to develop gout than those in the lowest quintile, whereas those who consumed the most seafood (both fish and shellfish) had a 51% higher risk than those who consumed the least.[5]

In addition to increasing incident gout risk, meat and seafood have also been shown to raise serum uric acid level. In the Third National Health and Nutrition Examination Survey (NHANES III), investigators surveyed the dietary habits of 14,809 participants and found that, after adjusting for age, the differences in uric acid levels between the top and bottom quintiles of consumption were 0.48 mg/dL (95% CI 0.34, 0.61; $P<.001$) for total meat and 0.16 mg/dL (95% CI 0.06, 0.27; $P = .005$) for seafood. After adjusting for several covariates, including age, sex, body mass index (BMI), serum creatinine, hypertension, alcohol use, and diuretic use, these differences remained statistically significant.[6]

Vegetables and Dairy

Consumption of vegetable and dairy protein appears to confer a protective effect against gout. In the HPFS, those in the highest quintile of vegetable protein intake were 27% less likely to develop gout than those in the lowest quintile, whereas top consumers of dairy protein had a 48% lower risk compared with those in the bottom fifth. Foods rich in vegetable and dairy protein tend to be low in purines, but even purine-rich plant foods (peas, beans, lentils, spinach, mushrooms, oatmeal, and cauliflower) were not associated with an increased risk of gout. The protective effect of dairy was limited to low-fat dairy products, but high-fat dairy products also did nothing to increase gout risk.[5]

In the NHANES III, those in the highest quintile of dairy consumption had a serum uric acid level 0.21 mg/dL lower than those in the lowest quintile (95% CI 0.04, 0.37; $P = .02$). Interestingly, those who consumed milk once or more per day had a lower serum uric acid level than those who did not (-0.25 mg/dL; 95% CI -0.40, -0.09 and $P<.001$), whereas those who consumed yogurt at least once every other day had a lower serum uric acid level than those who did not (-0.26 mg/dL; 95% CI -0.41, -0.12; $P<.001$).[6] These findings closely parallel those in the HPFS and provide strong evidence for the observed trends in incident gout risk in that study.

Alcohol

The HPFS also demonstrated a strong association between alcohol intake and an increased risk of gout. The degree of association grew as the level of consumption increased and varied with the type of beverage. Specifically, consumption of beer showed the strongest link, with a relative risk of 1.49 (95% CI 1.32–1.70) per 12 ounce serving per day. Consumption of liquor was also significantly associated with gout, with a relative risk of 1.15 (95% CI 1.04–1.28) per drink or shot per day. Meanwhile, wine consumption was not associated with gout (relative risk 1.04; 95% CI 0.88–1.22).[7]

Beer, wine, and liquor intake also affects serum uric acid level. After adjusting for other risk factors for hyperuricemia and consumption of the other alcoholic beverages surveyed, the NHANES III found that both beer (0.46 mg/dL per serving per day; 95% CI 0.32, 0.60) and liquor (0.29 mg/mL per serving per day; 95% CI 0.14, 0.45) increased serum uric acid level, whereas wine (0.04 mg/mL per serving per day;

95% CI −0.20, 0.11) did not.[8] These findings corroborate earlier studies linking gout attacks to alcohol consumption[9] but suggest that nonalcoholic components may play an important role. For instance, beer has a large purine content, whereas wine and liquor do not. The ingested purine in beer, in combination with the hyperuricemic effect of the alcohol itself, may account for its stronger association with gout. It is not known whether any protective effects of wine account for its lack of a demonstrable gout risk.[10]

Fructose

Another dietary factor that deserves special mention given its widespread consumption is fructose. According to the HPFS, men who consume increased amounts of sugar-sweetened soft drinks and other sources of fructose, including fruit juice and fructose-rich fruits like apples or oranges, have an increased risk of gout. Specifically, those who consumed two or more servings of sugar-sweetened soft drinks per day were 85% more likely to develop gout than those who drank less than one per month. Diet drinks, by contrast, were not associated with any increased risk.[11] Similarly, the NHANES III showed higher serum uric acid levels with increasing consumption of sugar-sweetened soft drinks. Drinking the equivalent of 0.5 to 0.9 servings per day increased serum uric acid level by 0.15 mg/dL, whereas drinking 1.0 to 3.9 servings per day increased the level by 0.33 mg/dL (95% CI 0.11, 0.73; $P<.001$ for trend). Consumption of diet soft drinks was not associated with any increase in serum uric acid levels.[12]

Coffee and Tea

By contrast, coffee consumption is associated with a decreased risk of gout. As the number of daily cups of coffee increases, the risk of incident gout decreases. In the HPFS, the multivariate relative risk associated with drinking no cups per day was 1.00, whereas for one to three daily cups it was 0.92, and for four to five cups it was 0.60 (95% CI 0.41–0.87, $P = .009$). Decaffeinated coffee showed a modest inverse association with gout, whereas tea intake and total daily caffeine intake showed no protective effect.[13] Serum uric acid level also decreases with increasing coffee intake, lower by 0.26 mg/dL (95% CI 0.11, 0.41) for those drinking four to five cups daily and 0.43 mg/dL (95% CI 0.23, 0.65) for those drinking six or more cups daily compared with those who do not drink coffee ($P<.001$). Similarly, decaffeinated coffee intake has a modest inverse association with uric acid level, whereas tea and total caffeine intake have no effect. These findings suggest components of coffee other than caffeine may play a role in reducing the risk of hyperuricemia and gout. Potential mechanisms include a possible link between antioxidants in coffee and decreased insulin levels. Insulin decreases renal excretion of urate, and insulin resistance is associated with hyperuricemia.[14]

Obesity

Common comorbidities should be considered in any discussion of lifestyle and dietary modifications for patients with gout. In addition to data on dietary risk factors, the HPFS reported findings linking gout to obesity. Those men with an elevated BMI had an increased relative risk of developing gout compared with those who were of normal weight. Those who had gained 30 or more pounds since age 21 were 1.99 times more likely to develop gout than those who maintained their weight (95% CI, 1.49–2.66). Meanwhile, losing 10 or more pounds during the course of the study had a protective effect (relative risk 0.61; 95% CI, 0.40–0.92).[15] Other studies have linked gout and hyperuricemia to the metabolic syndrome with a prevalence of 63%

among gout patients compared with 25% among patients without gout.[16] Gout has also been linked with diabetes mellitus,[17] cardiovascular disease,[18] and even mortality.[19] Given these findings, gout should itself be considered an important risk factor for metabolic diseases. Consequently, any lifestyle or dietary intervention for gout should simultaneously target these associated "lifestyle" diseases in an effort to minimize risk. Unfortunately, recent data indicate that patients with gout are not routinely following evidence-based dietary recommendations.[20]

Summary

Gout is an inflammatory arthritis associated with several dietary and lifestyle risk factors. Meat, seafood, and sugar-sweetened beverages increase the risk of gout, as do beer and liquor, but not wine. By contrast, vegetable proteins, low-fat dairy products, and coffee decrease the risk of gout. Because gout is associated with important chronic lifestyle-related diseases, including diabetes mellitus and the metabolic syndrome, dietary and lifestyle changes should address the increased risk of those diseases. A reasonable approach should focus on daily exercise, weight control, and limiting intake of fructose and refined carbohydrates as in patients with diabetes mellitus. Excessive intake of beer and liquor should be avoided, and dairy and vegetable proteins should replace some of those derived from meat and fish. Large prospective trials of such a diet in patients with gout are needed to determine the ability of diet and lifestyle modification to prevent gout recurrence.

OSTEOARTHRITIS AND DIET

Osteoarthritis (OA) is the most common form of arthritis and affects over 20 million individuals in the United States. Older age, female gender, obesity, history of trauma, repetitive use of joints, bone density, muscle weakness, and joint laxity all impact the development of OA.[21] Obesity remains one of the most important modifiable risk factors, and nonpharmacologic interventions, including weight loss and exercise, are the cornerstones of therapy.

Which Diet?

There are a variety of "fad diets" targeted to the general population despite a lack of scientific studies to support their various claims. Energy restrictive diets result in significant initial loss of bodyweight but are associated with high dropout and relapse-rates over time. Low-fat diets yield minimal success with respect to weight loss but do result in significantly lower blood lipid levels. High-protein, low-carbohydrate diets are advertised as the most effective at reducing bodyweight, although there has been no study comparing them to low-calorie diets for long-term weight loss.[22]

A study by Christensen and colleagues[23] examined the effectiveness of a rapid, diet-induced weight loss intervention on overweight individuals with OA of the knee. Eighty patients with knee OA, 89% of whom were women, were randomized either to a low-energy diet (LED) intervention (3.4 MJ/d) or a control diet (5 MJ/d). The LED intervention consisted of a nutritional powder that met recommendations for daily intake of high-quality protein and was taken as six daily meals. The control intervention consisted of a traditional hypoenergetic, high-protein, low-calorie diet taken in the form of ordinary foods based on recommendations from a nutritional advice session. At study conclusion, the LED group had lost more weight and body fat than the control group. There was also a greater decrease in Western Ontario and McMaster Universities Osteoarthritis Index (WOMAC) scores among the LED intervention group compared with the control group (mean between-groups difference 219.3 mm, $P = .005$). These results suggest that for OA patients a low-energy diet may be more beneficial than an ordinary diet because it yields more rapid weight loss and more significant loss of body fat.

The general recommendation for obese patients with OA is to adhere to a weight loss program with an initial goal of 10% body weight loss at a rate of 1 to 2 lb per week.[24] This has been shown to provide symptomatic relief and improve function by an average of 28%.[23] Regardless of the diet chosen, however, achieving and sustaining weight loss is difficult and requires a multidisciplinary team approach.

Inflammation and OA

Overweight individuals are at an increased risk of developing OA in weight-bearing joints. Although much of the risk is due to biomechanical factors, data suggest that other systemic effects may also play a role.[25,26] A number of studies have shown that decreasing body fat is more important than overall weight loss in improving symptoms. Adipose tissue serves as an endocrine organ and secretes a number of inflammatory markers, including leptin, tumor necrosis factor-alpha, and cytokines, that may mediate symptoms in OA through chronic inflammation.[27,28] Weight-loss programs for OA patients should therefore focus on loss of fat mass, particularly abdominal fat, while maintaining lean muscle mass.[29]

Exercise Programs

In combination with diet, exercise is another effective tool for weight loss and symptom reduction in OA. The Arthritis, Diet, and Activity Promotion Trial (ADAPT) was a randomized, single-blind clinical trial lasting 18 months designed to determine whether long-term exercise and dietary weight loss are effective, either separately or in combination, at improving functional impairment, pain, and mobility in older overweight individuals with OA of the knee. Three hundred and sixteen adults with knee OA and a BMI of at least 28 kg/m2 were recruited and randomized to one of four interventions: healthy lifestyle (control), diet only, exercise only, or diet plus exercise. The primary outcome was self-reported physical function using the WOMAC index. Secondary outcomes included weight loss, 6-minute walk distance, stair-climb time, WOMAC pain and stiffness scores, and changes in joint space width on radiographs of the knees. At study conclusion, the combination of dietary weight loss and exercise resulted in greater overall improvement in function and pain compared with control and with either intervention alone.[30]

Polyunsaturated Fatty Acids

Polyunsaturated fatty acids (PUFA) are classified as n-3, n-6, or n-9, depending on the position of the last double bond along the fatty acid chain. PUFAs are metabolized by cyclooxygenases (COX) and lipooxygenases (LOX) into different eicosanoids. The main dietary PUFAs are n-3-derived eicosanoids, which tend to be proinflammatory, and n-6-derived eicosanoids, which tend to be anti-inflammatory. Foods rich in omega-3 fatty acids include soybean, flaxseeds, walnuts, and fish and canola oils, whereas foods rich in omega-6 fatty acids include sunflower oil, soybean, safflower, corn, and meat. The modern Western diet is relatively low in n-3 PUFAs and high in n-6 PUFAs compared with the modern Eastern diet or the diet of preindustrial Western societies.[31]

High n-3 intake correlates with a decreased incidence of cardiovascular disease, but the role of anti-inflammatory fatty acids in OA is less clear.[32] A 24-week, double-blind, placebo-controlled trial of 10 mL daily cod liver oil supplementation (containing 786 mg of eicosapentaenoic acid) did not decrease the visual analog pain score or disability of 86 patients with a clinical diagnosis of OA.[33] In vitro, however, n-3 PUFAs have anti-inflammatory and anticatabolic properties based on their ability to decrease expression of aggrecanase, COX-2, 5-LOX-activating protein (5-LOX), 5-lip-oxygenase-activating protein (FLAP), interleukin-1 alpha (IL-1 alpha), tumor necrosis factor-α, matrix metalloproteinase (MMP)-3, and MMP-13.[34–36] At the same time, an imbalance of n-6 and n-3 may also be detrimental. Rats fed high doses of omega-3 fatty acids exhibited cartilage surface irregularities and localized proteoglycan depletion that may be similar to early changes seen in OA.[37]

Avocado and Soybean Unsaponifiables

Avocado and soybean unsaponifiables (ASU) are nutritional supplements widely used in Europe but, until recently, unavailable in the United States. In vitro, ASUs have anabolic and anti-inflammatory effects on chondrocytes.[38] A meta-analysis of four double-blind, randomized, placebo-controlled trials evaluated the effect of ASUs on knee and hip OA.[39] Two 3-month trials showed that 300 mg of ASUs once daily decreased nonsteroidal anti-inflammatory drug (NSAID) intake compared with placebo.[40,41] In a trial lasting 6 months, 300 mg of ASUs once daily showed an improved Lequesne functional index (LFI) compared with placebo. ASUs had a 2-month delayed onset of action with residual symptomatic effects up to 2 months after the end of treatment.[42] Although treatment with ASUs may improve symptoms, they have not been shown to have disease modifying capabilities. In a 2-year randomized, controlled trial (RCT) on hip OA, 300 mg of ASUs once daily did not slow the rate of joint space narrowing.[43] Furthermore, there was no effect on secondary endpoints (LFI, visual analog [VAS] of pain, NSAID intake, and patients' and investigators' global assessments) compared with placebo after 1 year. A post hoc analysis, however, did suggest that ASUs might decrease narrowing of joint space width in patients with severe hip OA. Thus, although some data suggest ASUs may be bring short-term symptomatic relief, their long-term effects and disease-modifying capabilities need further investigation.

Antioxidant Nutrients

Reactive oxygen species (ROS) play a crucial role in cartilage homeostasis through regulation of chondrocyte activities, including cell activation, proliferation, and matrix remodeling. When ROS are overproduced, as in OA, "oxidative stress" occurs, leading to structural and functional cartilage damage including cell death and matrix degradation.[44] Vitamin supplements, which have antioxidant properties, may therefore be beneficial in OA.

Vitamin C, or ascorbic acid, is a water-soluble antioxidant vitamin found in citrus fruits, rose hips, black currants, strawberries, Brussels sprouts, broccoli, peppers, cabbage, potatoes, and parsley. The Framingham Osteoarthritis Cohort Study showed that a moderate intake of vitamin C (120–200 mg/d) was associated with a threefold reduction in risk of OA progression compared with low vitamin C intake.[45] A multicenter, randomized, double-blind, placebo-controlled case-crossover study of 133 patients with hip or knee OA showed that 1 g of calcium ascorbate (containing 898 mg vitamin C) taken twice daily was more effective in decreasing pain than placebo.[38] Determining the safety of using such high doses of vitamin C, however, requires further long-term data.

Vitamin E is found in vegetable and nut oils, safflower oil, nuts, sunflower seeds, and whole grains. Five randomized clinical trials have been conducted to assess the benefit of vitamin E in the symptomatic treatment of OA. Two trials concluded that Vitamin E was more effective than placebo in decreasing pain.[46,47] A third suggested that Vitamin E was as effective as diclofenac.[48] Two more recent studies performed over a longer period, however, showed no benefit. A 6-month double-blind RCT of 500 IU of vitamin E daily in 77 patients showed no improvement in pain, stiffness, or physical function compared with placebo.[49] Similarly, a 2-year double-blind RCT of 500 IU of vitamin E daily in 136 patients showed no symptomatic or structure-modifying benefit over placebo.[50] Thus, although vitamin E may be beneficial for short-term symptomatic relief of OA, its utility in long-term symptomatic treatment is less clear.

Summary

OA is a chronic degenerative disorder and a source of pain and functional impairment for millions of patients. Weight loss and exercise are the mainstays of treatment and, in combination, result in significant improvement of function and pain. Of the various dietary programs used by patients, diets focusing on the loss of fat mass are the most beneficial. Dietary supplements like ASUs and antioxidant nutrients have been shown to decrease pain in some, but not all, studies. More prospective clinical trials are needed to elucidate their role in the management of OA.

RHEUMATOID ARTHRITIS AND DIET

Dietary manipulation has been used for symptomatic treatment of rheumatoid arthritis (RA) since the 1920s, although it was met with skepticism by a large majority of physicians.[51] In the past 2 decades, more studies have emerged looking at the effects of dietary modification on rheumatic disease. The possible benefits of dietary therapy are thought to arise from alteration in gut flora, reduction in permeability to bacteria and other antigens, and elimination of offending foods.[29]

Mediterranean Diet

The Mediterranean diet is high in plant foods (fruits, vegetables, cereals, beans, nuts, seeds), fish, and olive oil, and low in red meat.[52] Skoldstam and colleagues[53] conducted a randomized clinical trial of 56 patients comparing a 12-week Cretan Mediterranean diet, which features olive oil as the principal fat as well as moderate wine consumption, with an ordinary diet. After 12 weeks, there was a significant difference in pain VAS in favor of the intervention group (mean difference −14.00; 95% CI −23.63,−4.37). There was a nonsignificant difference in physical function health assessment questionnaire (HAQ) score, although there was a significant change from baseline to follow up in favor of the intervention group. There was also a nonsignificant difference in morning stiffness in favor the Mediterranean diet group. Overall, patients in the intervention group had a reduction in disease activity score using 28 joint counts (DAS28) and an increase in physical function and vitality as measured by the Short Form-36 Health Survey (SF-36).[53]

A second, controlled Mediterranean-diet intervention trial was conducted by McKellar and colleagues[54] in 2007 with a total of 130 patients. The intervention group attended weekly 2-hour sessions, including hands-on cooking classes reinforced with written information, while the control group was given written dietary information only. There was significant improvement in VAS pain scores in the intervention group at 3 and 6 months follow-up. There was also a significant improvement in physical function HAQ score at 3 months and improvement in morning stiffness at 6 months in those on the Mediterranean diet.

Vegetarian Diet

Vegetarian diets for patients with RA have gained increased publicity in recent years. It has been postulated that in addition to helping patients maintain a healthy weight, a vegetarian diet rich in fruits and vegetables and low in saturated fat may decrease total body inflammation by altering levels of arachidonic acid, antioxidants, and essential fatty acids, and by reducing food antigens.[55,56]

In a randomized, single-blind trial of 53 patients with RA, subjects in the experimental group underwent a vegetable juice fast for 7 to 10 days followed by a vegan diet for 3.5 months. The vegan diet excluded gluten, refined sugar, citrus fruits, meat, fish, eggs, dairy products, alcohol, coffee, tea, salt, strong spices, and preservatives. The patients were then transitioned to a lacto-vegetarian diet for 9 months, and milk, dairy products, and gluten were reintroduced into the diet every second day. If patients experienced pain, stiffness, or joint swelling within 2 to 48 hours of food reintroduction, the food was eliminated for at least 7 days. The patients were then rechallenged with the food item, and if symptoms returned, the food item was excluded from their diet for the remainder of the study. The control group consumed an ordinary diet throughout the entire study. After 4 weeks, the diet group showed significant improvement in all clinical variables, including tender and swollen joints, pain, duration of morning stiffness, grip strength, and changes in overall health assessment compared with controls.[57] At 1 year follow-up, patients who initially showed improvement (diet responders) continued to have improved symptoms compared with both diet nonresponders and the control group. Furthermore, all diet responders and half of the nonresponders at follow-up continued to maintain a modified diet of either the original lacto-vegetarian study diet or an omnivorous diet excluding foods thought to exacerbate their symptoms. The investigators concluded that some patients with RA may benefit from a vegetarian diet, and this diet may be a useful supplement to conventional treatment.

Elimination Diet

Elimination diets remove food items thought to trigger symptoms. These foods are then slowly reintroduced in hopes of identifying those that cause a real change in disease activity. The most common food intolerances are corn, wheat, bacon or pork, oranges, milk, oats, rye, eggs, beef, and coffee.[58] Some believe that food antigens found in these and other foods play a role in the pathogenesis of rheumatic disease and that their elimination from the diet can cause symptom improvement.[59] In a single-blind, placebo-controlled crossover study, Darlington and colleagues[60] compared an elimination diet with an ordinary diet in 53 patients with RA. All patients underwent a 2-week washout period in which previous therapy was withdrawn. Patients were then randomly assigned to either immediate dietary therapy or placebo for 6 weeks followed by the elimination diet. Foods least likely to cause intolerance were reintroduced first in a stepwise manner, followed by foods that more often cause intolerance, such as cereals. Any foods producing symptoms of RA were removed from the diet. At study conclusion, there was significant objective improvement during dietary therapy for all measured variables including pain, duration of morning stiffness, number of painful joints, grip strength, and time to walk 20 yards. Of the 44 patients who completed the trial, 33 felt "better" or "much better" on a five-point scale after completing dietary treatment.

Elemental Diet

An elemental diet is a hypoallergenic, protein-free, artificial diet consisting of the simplest formulations of essential amino acids, glucose, medium-chain triglycerides, vitamins, and minerals. It is commercially manufactured as a powdered drink mix and can be used to replace one or more meals. Kavanagh and colleagues[59] assessed the effects of an elemental diet compared with a control diet in 47 patients with RA for

4 weeks. At study completion there was a statistically significant improvement in grip strength and Ritchie score in the diet group, although improvement was not sustained upon food reintroduction. Furthermore, there was a high dropout rate, as only 38% of patients initially enrolled in the study completed the trial.

In a second study by Holst-Jensen and colleagues,[61] 30 patients were randomized to either a liquid, elemental-diet or continuation of a normal diet. Outcome measures included pain intensity, morning stiffness, HAQ-score, number of swollen joints, joint tenderness, erythrocyte sedimentation rate, and the patient's global assessment of health. At the end of the 4 week study, there was significant improvement in the average level of pain and HAQ-score of those on the elemental diet, but the effects were transient and no longer present at 3 and 6 months follow-up.

Summary

Dietary manipulation may improve symptoms in a subset of RA patients, but these diets are often associated with a high dropout rate. Proposed mechanisms of improvement include altered antioxidant levels, weight loss, and removal of food allergens and intolerances. The improvement of symptoms seen in clinical studies may also be due to change from an unhealthy diet to a healthier diet with increased consumption of fruits and vegetables and a reduction of saturated fats during the course of the study. The effects of dietary manipulation require further randomized, long-term studies to confirm the benefits of specific diets before specific recommendations can be made.

FIBROMYALGIA AND DIET

Fibromyalgia is a common cause of chronic widespread musculoskeletal pain, diffuse tenderness, and fatigue. Its cause is unknown, but it is thought to be due to altered central nervous system pain processing. According to surveys of patients with fibromyalgia, many believe their symptoms are affected by dietary intake. In one study, 42% of patients reported exacerbation of symptoms such as pain, stiffness, and joint swelling after intake of certain foods.[62] In another, 68% used nutritional supplements in an attempt to control symptoms.[63] Despite the belief that diet may play a role in the pathophysiology and, by extension, the treatment of fibromyalgia, supportive data to that effect is lacking. Existing studies are hampered by methodological limitations and the absence of plausible biologic mechanisms.

A recent review has summarized available data regarding fibromyalgia and diet.[64] Only nine studies enrolled patients using standard criteria for fibromyalgia and tested dietary intervention. Of these, one was a prospective, randomized, controlled trial, and two were nonrandomized, controlled trials. The remainder were observational or descriptive studies. No studies have identified specific foods or additives that appear to cause or exacerbate fibromyalgia. To date, dietary intervention studies for fibromyalgia have focused on vegetarian, weight loss, or elimination diets.

Vegetarian and Vegan Diets

Azad and colleagues[65] conducted a randomized, controlled crossover trial comparing the effects of a vegetarian diet versus amitriptyline for treatment of fatigue, insomnia, pain, and tenderness in 78 patients with fibromyalgia. On all counts, the amitriptyline cohort fared better, with greater, statistically significant relief of symptoms. Patients on a vegetarian diet had no significant change in symptoms except for pain score, though the difference was less than that observed in the amitriptyline group. At the end of a 6 week observational period, all patients in the vegetarian arm of the trial discontinued the diet in favor of amitriptyline.

Three studies tested raw vegetarian or vegan diets rich in antioxidants and composed primarily of vegetables, fruits, berries, seeds, and nuts with avoidance of alcohol, caffeine, meat, and dairy. One controlled study of 33 patients with fibromyalgia showed a significant decrease in self-reported morning stiffness and pain at rest compared with controls after 3 months.[66] The second found that 18 self-selected participants had significantly improved pain, sleep quality, and morning stiffness, as well as decreased BMI and serum cholesterol compared with 15 patients on an omnivorous diet. However, it is unclear whether weight loss or dietary changes were responsible for improved symptoms, a question beyond the study's design and statistical analysis.[67] Additionally, in both studies all patients voluntarily returned to an omnivorous diet at the conclusion of the 3 month study periods. The third study showed significant improvements in Fibromyalgia Impact Questionnaire, SF-36, quality of life survey, shoulder pain, flexibility, and 6-minute walk test, among other measures, in 18 subjects who completed the 7-month study. Despite these positive results, conclusions were limited by small sample size, a lack of control group, and participation of the patients in a motivational presentation which may have confounded results. Of note, although all subjects had previously been diagnosed with fibromyalgia by a rheumatologist, not all met diagnostic criteria at the time of trial entry.[68]

Weight Loss

Given available data, it is unclear whether obesity increases the occurrence or severity of fibromyalgia. A survey of 211 women with fibromyalgia, of whom 32% were obese, showed a correlation between BMI and the HAQ score (measuring the ability to perform activities of daily living), fatigue, and the number of tender points but could not conclude that symptoms of fibromyalgia are either due to obesity or responsive to weight loss.[69] Nonrandomized, uncontrolled studies of behavioral weight loss and surgical weight loss by gastric bypass have shown improvement in symptoms of fibromyalgia, body satisfaction, and quality of life associated with significant weight reduction.[70,71] However, without controls it is not clear whether symptomatic improvement can be attributed to weight loss itself rather than concurrent increases in physical activity, healthier diet, or supportive counseling.

Elimination Diets

In a study by Deuster and Jaffe,[72] 51 patients with fibromyalgia self-selected into treatment or control groups. A lymphocyte response assay was used to determine food sensitivities in the treatment group and revealed the most commonly reactive substances to be monosodium glutamate, caffeine, food coloring, chocolate, shrimp, dairy products, and aspartame. Treatment patients were asked to exclude foods to which they were sensitive and replace them with dietary supplements, including antioxidants, minerals, and other substances. Control patients continued their normal diets, while all subjects participated in biweekly support group meetings. At study conclusion, nearly half of the treatment group had dropped out due to lack of program adherence, but the remainder experienced less pain, depression, fatigue, and stiffness after 3 months compared with baseline. Significant drawbacks to these findings, however, include a failure to report control data and statistical significance as well as a lack of further improvement at the 6 month interval. Because of the nonrandomized, nonblinded design, significant dropout rate, and simultaneous dietary elimination, supplementation, and support group participation, it is impossible to draw firm conclusions from this study.

Despite the generally poor quality and inconclusive results of trials to date, focused elimination diets may yet deserve further study.[64] Central nervous system sensitization is one mechanism thought to be involved in dysfunctional pain processing in patients with fibromyalgia. Glutamate and aspartate, amino acids found in meat, monosodium glutamate, aspartame, and other food additives, are excitatory neurotransmitters which may contribute to central sensitization and play a role in the perception of pain in patients with fibromyalgia. Indeed, some have shown a correlation between glutamate levels in cerebrospinal fluid and the brain and pain levels in fibromyalgia.[73,74] Although these data do not show causality, some suggest that dietary intake of these neurotransmitter amino acids may play a role in pain perception in some patients with fibromyalgia. A case series of four patients with fibromyalgia did report complete or nearly complete resolution of symptoms with dietary exclusion of monosodium glutamate and aspartame and recurrence of symptoms with rechallenge.[75]

Summary

With limited available data, one cannot yet draw definitive conclusions regarding the role of diet in fibromyalgia or make specific dietary recommendations for treatment. More rigorous, controlled trials of dietary intervention in fibromyalgia are warranted.

SUMMARY

Millions of people suffer from gout, OA, rheumatoid arthritis, and fibromyalgia. Each can be incapacitating and detrimental to quality of life. Although effective pharmacologic treatments are available for each, the continuing high burden of disease and lost productivity testifies to the need for further innovation. Diet, nutrition, and weight loss have shown promise in alleviating some of this disease burden, particularly in gout and OA. This type of lifestyle change may have the added benefit of giving patients a feeling of control and ownership over their disease as well as a nonpharmacologic means of treatment.

Unfortunately, many of the existing trials in this area suffer from a lack of methodological rigor, including the absence of suitable controls and randomization, confounding variables, high dropout rate, and short study duration. With these limitations, few definitive conclusions can be drawn. However, the role of diet in rheumatologic disease, particularly that of substances like antioxidants and omega-3 fatty acids which may decrease systemic inflammation, remains intriguing.

Future clinical studies should focus on promising basic science mechanisms and draw on an understanding of disease pathophysiology. Dietary intervention without plausible biologic mechanisms in mind is unlikely to be productive. Yet, by employing rigorous epidemiologic methods to basic biologic questions, as in the case of gout, important advances in understanding can be made. Ultimately, the role of diet, nutrition, and weight loss in rheumatologic disease is in many ways poorly-understood; yet, it remains intriguing and deserving of further study.

REFERENCES

1. Clifford AJ, Riumallo JA, Young VR, et al. Effects of oral purines on serum and urinary uric acid of normal, hyperuricaemic and gouty humans. J Nutr 1976; 106:428–50.
2. Emmerson BT. The management of gout. N Engl J Med 1996;334:445–51.
3. Fam AG. Gout, diet, and the insulin resistance syndrome. J Rheumatol 2002;29: 1350–5.

4. Dessein PH, Shipton EA, Stanwix AE, et al. Beneficial effects of weight loss associated with moderate calorie/carbohydrate restriction, and increased proportional intake of protein and unsaturated fat on serum urate and lipoprotein levels in gout: a pilot study. Ann Rheum Dis 2000;59:539–43.
5. Choi HK, Atkinson K, Karlson EW, et al. Purine-rich foods, dairy and protein intake, and the risk of gout in men. N Engl J Med 2004;350:1093–103.
6. Choi HK, Liu S, Curhan G. Intake of purine-rich foods, protein, dairy products, and serum uric acid level: the Third National Health and Nutrition Examination Survey. Arthritis Rheum 2005;52:283–9.
7. Choi HK, Atkinson K, Karlson EW, et al. Alcohol intake and risk of incident gout in men: a prospective study. Lancet 2004;363:1277–81.
8. Choi HK, Curhan G. Beer, liquor, wine, and serum uric acid level: the Third National Health and Nutrition Examination Survey. Arthritis Rheum 2004;51: 1023–9.
9. Gibson T, Rodgers AV, Simmonds HA, et al. A controlled study of diet in patients with gout. Ann Rheum Dis 1983;42:123–7.
10. Choia HK, Curhan G. Gout: epidemiology and lifestyle choices. Curr Opin Rheumatol 2005;17:341–5.
11. Choi HK, Curhan G. Soft drinks, fructose consumption, and the risk of gout in men: prospective cohort study. BMJ 2008;336:309–12.
12. Choi JW, Ford ES, Gao X, et al. Sugar-sweetened soft drinks, diet soft drinks, and serum uric acid level: the Third National Health and Nutrition Examination Survey. Arthritis Rheum 2008;59:109–16.
13. Choi HK, Willett W, Curhan G. Coffee, consumption and risk of incident gout in men: a prospective study. Arthritis Rheum 2007;56:2049–55.
14. Choi HK, Curhan G. Coffee, tea, and caffeine consumption and serum uric acid level: the Third National Health and Nutrition Examination Survey. Arthritis Rheum 2007;57:816–21.
15. Choi HK, Atkinson K, Karlson EW, et al. Obesity, weight change, hypertension, diuretic use, and risk of gout in men. Arch Intern Med 2005;165:742–8.
16. Choi HK, Ford ES, Li C, et al. Prevalence of the metabolic syndrome in patients with gout: the Third National Health and Nutrition Examination Survey. Arthritis Rheum 2007;57:109–15.
17. Choi HK, De Vera MA, Krishnan E. Gout and the risk of type 2 diabetes among men with a high cardiovascular risk profile. Rheumatology 2008;47:1567–70.
18. Krishnan E, Baker JF, Furst DE, et al. Gout and the risk of acute myocardial infarction. Arthritis Rheum 2006;54:2688–96.
19. Choi HK, Curhan G. Independent impact of gout on mortality and risk for coronary heart disease. Circulation 2007;116:894–900.
20. Shulten P, Thomas J, Miller M, et al. The role of diet in the management of gout: a comparison of knowledge and attitudes to current evidence. J Hum Nutr Diet 2009;22:3–11.
21. Zhang Y, Jordan JM. Epidemiology of osteoarthritis. Clin Geriatr Med 2010;26(3): 355–69.
22. Miller WC. Effective diet and exercise treatments for overweight and recommendations for intervention. Sports Med 2001;31(10):717–24.
23. Christensen R, Astrup A, Bliddal H. Weight loss: the treatment of choice for knee osteoarthritis? A randomized trial. Osteoarthr Cartil 2005;13(1):20–7.
24. National Institutes of Health. Clinical guidelines on the identification, evaluation, and treatment of overweight and obesity in adults-the evidence report. Obes Res 1998;6(2):51S–209S.

25. Sokoloff L, Mickelsen O. Dietary fat supplements, body weight and osteoarthritis in DBA/2JN mice. J Nutr 1965;85:117–21.
26. Sokoloff L, Michelsen O, Silverstein E, et al. Experimental obesity and osteoarthritis. Am J Physiol 1960;198:765–70.
27. Hauner H, Hochberg Z. Endocrinology of adipose tissue. Horm Metab Res 2002; 34:605–6.
28. Hauner H. Secretory factors from human adipose tissue and their functional role. Proc Nutr Soc 2005;64:163–9.
29. Rayman M. Dietary manipulation in musculoskeletal conditions. Best Pract Res Clin Rheumatol 2008;22(3):535–61.
30. Messier S, Loeser R, Miller G, et al. Exercise and dietary weight loss in overweight and obese older adults with knee osteoarthritis. The arthritis, diet, and activity promotion trial. Arthritis Rheum 2004;50(5):1501–10.
31. Ameye L, Chee W. Osteoarthritis and nutrition. From nutraceuticals to functional foods: a systematic review of the scientific evidence. Arthritis Res Ther 2006;8:R127.
32. Calder PC. n-3 Fatty acids and cardiovascular disease: evidence explained and mechanisms explored. Clin Sci (Lond) 2004;107:1–11.
33. Stanners T, Sibbald B, Freeling P. Efficacy of cod liver oil as an adjunct to non-steroidal anti-inflammatory drug treatment in the management of osteoarthritis in general practive. Ann Rheum Dis 1992;51:128–9.
34. Curtis CL, Hughes CE, Flannery CR, et al. n-3 fatty acids specifically modulate catabolic factors involved in articular cartilage degradation. J Biol Chem 2000; 275:721–4.
35. Curtis CL, Rees SG, Cramp J, et al. Effects of n-3 fatty acids on cartilage metabolism. Proc Nutr Soc 2002;61:381–9.
36. Curtis CL, Rees SG, Little CB, et al. Pathologic indications of degradation and inflammation in human osteoarthritic cartilage are abrogated by exposure to n-3 fatty acids. Arthritis Rheum 2002;46:1544–53.
37. Lippiello L, Fienhold M, Grandjean C. Metabolic and ultrastructural changes in articular cartilage of rats fed dietary supplements of omega-3 fatty acids. Arthritis Rheum 1990;33:1029–36.
38. Pablo P, Lo G, McAlindon T. Nutrition and nutritional supplements and osteoarthritis. In: Coleman LA, editor. Nutrition and rheumatic disease. Totowa (NJ): Humana Press; 2008. p. 128, 145.
39. Ernst E. Avocado-soybean unsaponifiables (ASU) for osteoarthritis—a systematic review. Clin Rheumatol 2003;22:285–8.
40. Blotman F, Maheu E, Wulwik A, et al. Efficacy and safety of avocado/soybean unsaponifiables in the treatment of symptomatic osteoarthritis of the knee and hip. A prospective, multicenter, three-month randomized, double-blind, placebo-controlled trial. Rev Rhum Engl Ed 1997;64(12):825–34.
41. Appelboom T, Schuermans J, Berbruggen G, et al. Symptoms modifying effect of avocado-soybean unsaponifiables (ASU) in knee osteoarthritis. A double blind, prospective, placebo-controlled study. Scand J Rheumatol 2001;30(4):242–7.
42. Maheu E, Mazieres B, Valat JP, et al. Symptomatic efficacy of avocado/soybean unsaponifiables in the treatment of osteoarthritis on the knee and hip: a prospective, randomized, double-blind, placebo-controlled, multicenter clinical trial with a six-month treatment period and a two-month followup demonstrating a persistent effect. Arthritis Rheum 1998;41(1):81–91.
43. Lequesne M, Maheu E, Cadet C, et al. Structural effect of avocado/soybean unsaponifiables on joint space loss in osteoarthritis of the hip. Arthritis Rheum 2002;47(1):50–8.

44. Henroitin Y, Kurz B, Aigner T. Oxygen and reactive oxygen species in cartilage degradation: friends or foes? Osteoarthr Cartil 2005;13(8):643–54.
45. McAlindon TE, Jacques P, Zhang Y, et al. Do antioxidant micronutrients protect against the development and progression of knee osteoarthritis? Arthritis Rheum 1996;39(4):648–56.
46. Machtey I, Ouaknine L. Tocopherol in osteoarthritis: a controlled pilot study. J Am Geriatr Soc 1978;26(7):328–30.
47. Blakenhorn G. Clinical effectiveness of Spondyvit (vitamin E) in activated arthroses. A multicenter placebo-controlled double-blind study. Z Orthop Ihre Grenzgeb 1986;124(3):340–3.
48. Scherak O, Kolarz G, Schodl C, et al. [High dosage vitamin E therapy in patients with activated arthrosis]. Z Rheumatol 1990;49(6):369–73 [in German].
49. Brand C, Snaddon J, Bailey M, et al. Vitamin E is ineffective for symptomatic relief of knee osteoarthritis: a six month double blind, randomized, placebo controlled study. Ann Rheum Dis 2001;60(10):946–9.
50. Wluka AE, Stuckey S, Brand C, et al. Supplementary vitamin E does not affect the loss of cartilage volume in knee osteoarthritis: a 2 year double blind randomized placebo controlled study. J Rheumatol 2002;29:2585–91.
51. McDougall J, Bruce B, Spiller G, et al. Effects of a very low-fat, vegan diet in subjects with rheumatoid arthritis. J Altern Complement Med 2002;8(1):71–5.
52. Rayman MP, Callaghan A. Nutrition and arthritis. Oxford: Blackwell Publishing; 2006.
53. Skoldstam L, Hagfors L, Johansson G. An experimental study of a Mediterranean diet intervention for patiets with rheumatoid arthritis. Ann Rheum Dis 2003;62(3): 208–14.
54. McKellar G, Morrison E, McEntegart A, et al. A pilot study of a Mediterranean-diet intervention in female patients with rheumatoid arthritis living in areas of social deprivation in Glasgow. Ann Rheum Dis 2007;66(9):1239–43.
55. Smedslund G, Byfuglien M, Olsen S, et al. Effectiveness and safety of dietary interventions for rheumatoid arthritis: a systematic review of randomized controlled trials. J Am Diet Assoc 2010;110(5):727–35.
56. Adam O, Beringer C, Kless T, et al. Anti-inflammatory effects of a low arachidonic acid diet and fish oil in patients with rheumatoid arthritis. Rheumatol Int 2003; 23(1):27–36.
57. Kjeldsen-Kragh J, Haugen M, Borchgrevink CF, et al. Controlled trial of fasting and one-year vegetarian diet in rheumatoid arthritis. Lancet 1991;338:899–902.
58. Darlington LG, Ramsey NW. Review of dietary therapy for rheumatoid arthritis. Br J Rheumatol 1993;32:507–14.
59. Kavanagh R, Workman E, Nash P, et al. The effects of elemental diet and subsequent food reintroduction on rheumatoid-arthritis. Br J Rheumatol 1995;34(3): 270–3.
60. Darlington LG, Ramsey NW, Mansfield JR. Placebo-controlled, blind study of dietary manipulation therapy in rheumatoid arthritis. Lancet 1986;1(8475):236–8.
61. Holst-Jensen SE, Pfeiffer-Jense M, Monsrud M, et al. Treatment of rheumatoid arthritis with a peptide diet: a randomized, controlled trial. Scand J Rheumatol 1998;27(5):329–36.
62. Haugen M, Kjeldsenkragh J, Nordvag BY, et al. Diet and disease symptoms in rheumatic diseases—results of a questionnaire based survey. Clin Rheumatol 1991;10(4):401–7.
63. Bennett R, Jones J, Turk DC, et al. An internet survey of 2,596 people with fibromyalgia. BMC Musculoskelet Disord 2007;8:27.

64. Holton KF, Kindler LL, Jones KD. Potential dietary links to central sensitization in fibromyalgia: past reports and future directions. Rheum Dis Clin North Am 2009; 35:409–20.

65. Azad KA, Alam MN, Haq SA, et al. Vegetarian diet in the treatment of fibromyalgia. Bangladesh Med Res Counc Bull 2000;26(2):41–7.

66. Hanninen, Kaartinen K, Rauma AL, et al. Antioxidants in vegan diet and rheumatic disorders. Toxicology 2000;155(1–3):45–53.

67. Kaartinen K, Lammi K, Hypen M, et al. Vegan diet alleviates fibromyalgia symptoms. Scand J Rheumatol 2000;29(5):308–13.

68. Donaldson MS, Speight N, Loomis S. Fibromyalgia syndrome improved using a mostly raw vegetarian diet: an observational study. BMC Complement Altern Med 2001;1:7.

69. Yunus MB, Arslan S, Aldag JC. Relationship between body mass index and fibromyalgia features. Scand J Rheumatol 2002;31(1):27–31.

70. Shapiro JR, Anderson DA, Danoff-Burg S. A pilot study of the effects of behavioral weight loss treatment on fibromyalgia symptoms. J Psychosom Res 2005;59(5):275–82.

71. Hooper MM, Stellato TA, Hallowell PT, et al. Musculoskeletal findings in obese subjects before and after weight loss following bariatric surgery. Int J Obes (Lond) 2007;31(1):114–20.

72. Deuster PA, Jaffe RM. A novel treatment for fibromyalgia improves clinical outcomes in a community-based study. J Muscoskel Pain 1998;6(2):133–49.

73. Larson AA, Giovengo SL, Russell IJ, et al. Changes in the concentrations of amino acids in the cerebrospinal fluid that correlate with pain in patients with fibromyalgia: implications for nitric oxide pathways. Pain 2000;87(2):201–11.

74. Harris RE, Sundgren PC, Pang Y, et al. Dynamic levels of glutamate within the insula are associated with improvements in multiple pain domains in fibromyalgia. Arthritis Rheum 2008;58(3):903–7.

75. Smith JD, Terpening CM, Schmidt SO, et al. Relief of fibromyalgia symptoms following discontinuation of dietary excitotoxins. Ann Pharmacother 2001;35(6): 702–6.

Index

Note: Page numbers of article titles are in **boldface** type.

A

Acupressure, for pediatric patients, 89
Acupuncture
    for pediatric patients, 88–89
    for SLE, 50
Alcohol intake, gout and, 120–121
Alternative medicine. *See* Complementary and alternative medicine.
Antiinflammatory effects
    of fish oil, 77–80
    of mindfulness meditation, 69–70
Antioxidants, for osteoarthritis, 124–125
Anxiety
    in fibromyalgia, 25–26
    in SLE, 48, 52
    mindfulness interventions for, 68–69
Arthralgia, in pediatric patients, 85–94
Arthritis, gouty, 119–122
Avocado-soybean unsaponifiables, for osteoarthritis, 96, 124
Ayurvedic medicine, for rheumatoid arthritis, 97–98

B

Back pain
    glucosamine for, 111
    herbal medicine for, 95–97
Behavioral therapy
    dialectical, 66–67
    for SLE, 51–52
Biofeedback, for pediatric patients, 89
Breathing exercises, for pediatric patients, 89

C

Calcium supplementation, for pediatric patients, 90
CAM. *See* Complementary and alternative medicine.
Cannabis, for rheumatoid arthritis, 98
Capsicum creams, for back pain, 96
Cardiovascular disorders, in rheumatoid arthritis, 23
Cartilage protection, glucosamine and chondroitin sulfate for, 103–118
Cat's claw, for rheumatoid arthritis, 98
Chinese herbal medicines, 97, 99
Chiropractic, for pediatric patients, 90–91

Rheum Dis Clin N Am 37 (2011) 135–142
doi:10.1016/S0889-857X(10)00114-6
0889-857X/11/$ – see front matter © 2011 Elsevier Inc. All rights reserved.

rheumatic.theclinics.com

Printed and bound by CPI Group (UK) Ltd, Croydon, CR0 4YY

03/10/2024

01040445-0012